Praise for *The Cure for Loneliness*

"Finally, a go-to guide for anyone struggling with loneliness and isolation. Dr. Bill Howatt inspires confidence, comfort, and a shared sense of purpose in this unique call to action. *The Cure for Loneliness* is the first book I've encountered that offers both a step-by-step path out of mental traps as well as a brightly lit path into positive relationships that will build and protect good mental health."

RYAN TODD, MD, FRCPC, CEO, *headversity*

"Dr. Bill Howatt offers useful, interesting exercises to assess your level of isolation and loneliness, as well as practical, impactful tips to get out of your mental trap. Not only does this book encourage every one of us to improve our resiliency, but it also inspires leaders to support their people and build a psychologically safe workplace."

RENÉE LÉGARÉ, MSc, ICD.D, PhD, executive VP and chief human resources officer, The Ottawa Hospital

"Learn the important difference between solitude, isolation, and loneliness—and more importantly, concrete ways of fending off their potential negative outcomes. Dr. Bill Howatt's real-life examples allow us to find hope in unexpected places."

LOUISE BRADLEY, CM, president and CEO, Mental Health Commission of Canada

"Read it, use it, feel better. Dr. Bill Howatt offers strategies to help you and those you lead reduce loneliness and improve mental health. An insightful and practical read."

STUART MACLEAN, CEO, Workers' Compensation Board of Nova Scotia

"Even if you're not especially lonely, you may still feel there's something missing in your life. Creating authentic connections can make all the difference. Enjoy this interesting read, but also use it to improve the quality of your life by freeing yourself from mental traps."

MARY ANN BAYNTON, MSW, principal, Mary Ann Baynton & Associates

"Dr. Bill Howatt is brilliant at explaining how our brain works and how we as human beings can unlock the mental traps that contribute to feelings of isolation and loneliness. This book is a must-read and a fantastic tool kit for anyone who wants to learn practical steps on how to deal with mental health barriers in order to increase our social connections and happiness."

MARIO BARIL, ombudsman for mental health and employee well-being, Innovation, Science and Economic Development Canada

"A must-read for anyone who senses their foundation of close friends and family is shifting under their feet. In my advocacy work on mental health at the political level, I knew change was taking place in our society and that our homes and workplaces were becoming lonelier places. Dr. Bill Howatt's book confirms this, but more importantly provides a pathway out of loneliness."

KEVIN FLYNN, Ontario minister of labour; chair, Ontario's Select Committee on Mental Health and Addictions

"*The Cure for Loneliness* provides practical tools for evaluating our social connections, and techniques for developing meaningful relationships in our personal and professional lives."

LYNN BROWNELL, president and CEO, Workplace Safety & Prevention Services

"*The Cure for Loneliness* gives us the wisdom to understand why connecting is so important. Dr. Bill Howatt offers a practical tool kit for forming authentic connections with friends, family, and communities. Reading this book brought me a deep understanding of how social media can deceive us into thinking that we have an abundance of friends and connections, when we are actually starving ourselves of true human connection."

SANDRA BOYD, SVP and national practice leader of career transition and career management, Optimum Talent

The Cure for Loneliness

The Cure for Loneliness

HOW TO FEEL CONNECTED
AND ESCAPE ISOLATION

Dr. Bill Howatt

PAGE TWO
BOOKS

Copyright © 2021 by Dr. William A. Howatt

All rights reserved. No part of this book may be reproduced, stored in a retrieval system or transmitted, in any form or by any means, without the prior written consent of the publisher or a licence from The Canadian Copyright Licensing Agency (Access Copyright). For a copyright licence, visit accesscopyright.ca or call toll free to 1-800-893-5777.

Some names and identifying details have been changed to protect the privacy of individuals.

This book is not intended as a replacement for therapy or as a substitute for the medical advice of physicians; it's designed to leverage techniques that can promote positive mental health. The reader should regularly consult a physician in matters relating to their health and particularly with respect to any symptoms that may require diagnosis or medical attention. The exercises in this book leverage the cognitive-behavioural approach. If engaging in any of these exercises creates more stress and strain, stop and seek professional support (e.g., call your local mental health agency, crisis line, employee and family assistance office, or 911).

Cataloguing in publication information is available from Library and Archives Canada.
ISBN 978-1-77458-000-4 (paperback)
ISBN 978-1-77458-056-1 (ebook)

Page Two
pagetwo.com

Edited by Amanda Lewis and Al Kingsbury
Copyedited by Crissy Calhoun
Proofread by Alison Strobel
Cover design by Taysia Louie
Interior design by Setareh Ashrafologhalai
Printed and bound in Canada by Friesens
Distributed in Canada by Raincoast Books
Distributed in the US and internationally by Publishers Group West, a division of Ingram

21 22 23 24 25   5 4 3 2 1

billhowatt.com

To all my authentic connections (ACs),
you know who you are

To my mom, whom I lost during the COVID-19 pandemic
and who helped me face the challenges of life

To LMN, who inspired me to write this
book and is one of my most significant ACs

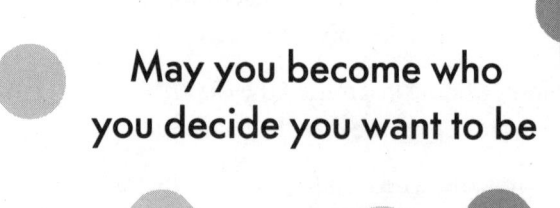

May you become who
you decide you want to be

Contents

Introduction 1

I The Anatomy of Isolation and Loneliness

1. Establish the Baseline of Your Relationships 13
2. Understand Isolation and Loneliness 17
3. What Causes Social Connections Gaps? 29
4. The Connection Between Technology and Loneliness 33

II Escaping the Mental Trap

5. How Mental Traps Form 43
6. How to Boost Resiliency 71
7. Framing to Unlock Your Mental Trap 109
8. Unlocking the Mental Trap 123

III How to Build Authentic Connections

9. The Path to Authentic Connections 133
10. Build Authentic Connections with Intention 159
11. Loneliness in the Workplace: A Guide for Employers 183

Conclusion 195

Acknowledgements 197

Notes 199

Index 211

Introduction

You never let a serious crisis go to waste. And what I mean by that is it's an opportunity to do things you think you could not do before.
RAHM EMANUEL

ON MARCH 12, 2020, I was in Edmonton to give a talk on psychological safety in the workplace. The threat of COVID-19 was increasing, and engagement cancellations started. Within hours, many of my speaking events for the coming weeks were off my calendar. I was in disbelief. Within a few days, all my talks for April and May were cancelled.

My employer, the Conference Board of Canada (CBOC), moved quickly to respond to the pandemic. We decided to start working remotely, and we created a COVID-19 landing page to share economic insights, relevant research, and my mental health video blog. Being an expert in mental health, I wanted to help people get through this crisis.

Canadians began learning the importance of social distancing and social isolation. I never liked the term "social distancing." In fact, in one of my early video blogs I called it "physical distancing" because while we wanted people to stay apart, we wanted them to stay connected socially.

On March 20, after five days in isolation in my townhouse in Ottawa, the magnitude of what was happening hit me. I was witnessing so much fear and concern around isolation and loneliness. I didn't go to bed with a plan, but when I woke up, I made a commitment to write this book. There's nothing like a pandemic to clarify a need for action.

Before COVID-19, isolation and loneliness were already challenges for a significant percentage of the population. In 2019, studies reported that one in five Canadians identified as lonely.[1] University of Chicago professor John Cacioppo suggested in an interview in *The Atlantic* that around 28 percent of the US population is experiencing loneliness, and it appears this number has grown by about 3 to 7 percent over the last 20 years.[2] Part of the loneliness epidemic lies in the fact that more people are choosing to live alone as they move to urban areas for work and education. The number of persons living alone in Canada more than doubled over 35 years, from 1.7 million in 1981 to 4 million in 2016.[3] Now that doesn't mean all these people are feeling socially disconnected, isolated, or lonely. But the social isolation of the COVID-19 pandemic further tested already strained social connections. An Ipsos poll reported that during the first month of the pandemic, 54 percent of Canadians responded that physical distancing left them feeling lonely or isolated.[4]

All humans have a genetic need to be socially connected, and we benefit from all types of social connections from informal to formal, from a simple smile from a stranger at a grocery store to a hug from a relative or close friend. All social connections, whether slight or intimate, help us feel connected to other humans.

We hear a lot about maintaining relationships, but what if relationship management is not the biggest social connection problem? Perhaps it's the absence of meaningful social connections in the first place.

What matters is that we value our social connections. When we don't have social connections we value, we have social connections gaps. Those gaps result in feelings of isolation and loneliness.

The Effects of Loneliness

Authentic connections are grounded in mutual respect, where both parties benefit. It's these types of relationships, when built into our personal and professional lives, that provide a feeling of social connection. The more authentic connections we have, the less likely we'll experience gaps in social connections. However, having just one authentic connection can mean the difference between happiness and loneliness.[5] Research suggests that the bonds of authentic connections are a major factor in predicting happiness.[6] Authentic connections can also improve our health: 148 independent studies that included more than 300,000 participants found that greater social connection is associated with a 50 percent reduction in risk of early death.[7]

When a person perceives they're socially isolated and lonely, their mental health and well-being are strained. There's evidence that links a lack of social support to poor mental health, as well as poor physical health outcomes, including cancer and infectious diseases.[8] Julianne Holt-Lunstad and colleagues reported that lacking social connections carries a risk factor that may exceed the risk of smoking up to 15 cigarettes a day, obesity, physical inactivity, or air pollution.[9]

Loneliness has been linked to depression, anxiety, irritability, and even suicide.[10] Sarah Pressman of the University of California, Irvine, demonstrated that while obesity reduces longevity by 20 percent, drinking by 30 percent, and smoking by 50 percent, loneliness reduces longevity by a whopping 70 percent.[11] Another study found that loneliness increases the chance of stroke or coronary heart disease, the leading cause of death in developed countries, by 30 percent.[12]

As I researched the effects of social connections gaps, I discovered lots of papers on the negative impact that isolation and loneliness can have on the population. The United Kingdom created a Minister for Loneliness position because of the research linking loneliness to premature death.[13] According to the Jo Cox Commission on Loneliness, more than 9 million people in Britain, around 14 percent of the population, often feel lonely, and it's estimated this costs employers £3.5 billion annually.[14]

A person experiencing loneliness can be more distracted, which may put them at increased risk of:

- Accidents
- Forgetfulness
- Failure to follow through on commitments
- Difficulty concentrating
- Difficulty relaxing

Interestingly, these risks are also found in a person experiencing high levels of stress. Loneliness is stressful. The absence of meaningful social connections in your family, community, and work life can be painful. Whether experienced in one or all areas of life, loneliness can create challenges that strain your mental health.

"I believe a lot of disease comes from anxiety, loneliness."

TOM COCHRANE

Simply put, social connections are good for our health. Learning to close social connections gaps and build social connections with people you feel psychologically safe around and share experiences with will support your mental health in particular.[15]

If you want to bake a cake, you require specific ingredients. If you want to bake happiness into your life, you need strong and healthy social connections. Think about it: If you could close one social connections gap immediately, which one would it be? Why did you pick this one, and what do you believe it will give you?

Sometimes a person may not be able to even name what they're experiencing as isolation or loneliness. All they know is they don't feel good or happy. The COVID-19 pandemic has a silver lining: it brought social connections gaps, isolation, and loneliness into the mainstream conversation. Education is important, and the more we can talk about isolation and loneliness, the more we can all learn what it is and what we can do about it.

Four Pillars for Mental Health

Most people know the simple formula for success in physical health. If you want to lose weight, for instance, you need to increase your exercise and decrease your caloric intake. What's left is making a free choice to value and do those actions that promote good physical health. The same is true for promoting your mental health.

In my work prior to the COVID-19 pandemic, I spent a lot of energy focusing on resiliency and coping skills. In my talks, I showed what stress and strained mental health look like in the workplace in particular and offered strategies for escaping the ruts that keep us stuck. Thinking about social connections' impact, I created a model for mental health, consisting of four pillars:

Physical health: What we put in our mouth impacts our brain chemistry, and the amount of sleep we get and the amount of physical activity we engage in affects our mood. Lifestyle choices, such as drinking or drug use, also impact our mental health.

Mental fitness: I believe that teaching prosocial coping skills and resiliency can help people improve their mental health. It is possible to assess which areas of our life could gain from enhanced attention and care, as I showed in my previous book, *Stop Hiding and Start Living*.[16] Organizations also play a role in supporting employees' resiliency by paying attention to what they're doing that's positively or negatively impacting their experience and closing expectation gaps to reduce stress and strain.

Social connections: One way to mitigate our risk of isolation and loneliness is to increase the number of our quality social connections. By forming and maintaining authentic connections and social safety networks, we are able to close the gaps where isolation and loneliness creep in.

Environmental factors: Income; education level; employment; access to food, housing, and health care; disability; ethnicity; gender; and psychological health and safety in the workplace all are factors that can contribute to mental health. Ultimately, our mental health is defined by what we do with and our experience in our environment.

How to Use This Book

I live with attention deficit hyperactivity disorder (ADHD), visual and auditory learning disability, and anxiety. I've seen first-hand that the quality of a person's social connections can predict their risk of mental illness and addictive disorders, such as substance abuse and pathological gambling.

As a behavioural scientist with 30-plus years' experience in helping people build their mental health, I know that setting up the conditions for change is half the battle, and sometimes you don't know where to start. But I know who does the work and makes the change: it's always the client. In fact, it's common practice for me to set expectations up front in counselling. I let the client know I don't do the work; they do. All I do is facilitate a new beginning by sharing information and examples, asking self-reflection questions, recommending exercises, supporting them to build a personalized action plan, and encouraging them to achieve their goals. Most of the change happens outside our one-hour weekly therapy sessions. That's where this book comes in, as a resource for you and a pathway forward.

In Part I, I'll break down the anatomy of isolation and loneliness, and I'll show how digital connections can be helpful but aren't a replacement for in-person support and camaraderie. I'll explain how to find the baseline of your relationships, so you know where you're at in terms of connecting with others.

One common challenge to developing social connections is when we perceive barriers to building or maintaining these connections. In Part II, I'll show you how and why we get stuck in the thinking ruts I call mental traps. Plainly put, negative thoughts, beliefs, and feelings limit our ability to close social connections gaps. The more our mental trap runs automatic negative thinking, the less likely we are to try to change, whether it's asking for support from our social connections or helping others we care about. I'll show you how a tried and true cognitive-behavioural approach (CBA) can assist in removing barriers to social connections.

Finally, in Part III, I'll give you a range of exercises that show you how to build authentic connections in your life, both personal and professional. No single pill or exercise offers an escape from isolation; the cure for loneliness lies in a combination of realizing where you're stuck and closing social connections gaps in meaningful ways.

The Cure for Loneliness

It's possible to feel isolated and not lonely, or lonely and not isolated. However, in this book, I'll examine the interdependencies of these two issues, as for the most part I see them correlated—meaning if you have a high perception of isolation, you're more likely to be at higher risk of loneliness. In a study I did in partnership with the *Globe and Mail* and Workplace Safety & Prevention Services (WSPS) Ontario on isolation and loneliness, we found evidence to suggest employees who reported higher perceived isolation typically also reported higher levels of loneliness.[17] We also found that employees with higher levels of resiliency on average had lower levels of perceived isolation and loneliness.

You don't need to be experiencing isolation and loneliness to benefit from this book. You may be struggling to find the quality of social connections you want, or perhaps have some confidence issues in getting the kinds of social connections you need.

Keep in mind that establishing or improving social connections is a process. Doing a bit every day can help strengthen your social connections muscle, which like any muscle will get stronger if you train it carefully and with patience. With hope and self-awareness, you can form new social connections you may not have believed possible. Success will happen, one step at a time.

After years of providing counselling, I've learned that many times a client is hyper-focused on their own world, which makes sense. They don't realize that I may have seen someone in the same kind of situation before and know the journey from where they are to light. With light come motivation and commitment to finding a new way of living. I tell clients that I love my job because I know where the light switch is. The client only needs to believe there's light. It's my job to help them see it. Once they see the light and change their perspective, we're ready to begin.

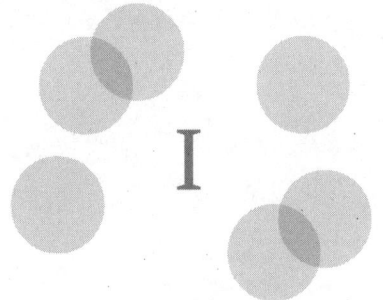

I

The Anatomy of Isolation and Loneliness

1

Establish the Baseline of Your Relationships

LET'S START by figuring out how fulfilling your current social connections are by establishing the baseline of your relationships.

Because social connections are good for our mental health, our perceived benefit of our social connections predicts our mental health. For example, the higher your perceived benefit, the more satisfied you are with your social connections. Now, what is important to keep in mind as you complete this exercise is that no one relationship can meet 100 percent of your needs. As well, keep in mind that it is difficult to have meaningful relationships with others if you do not have peace within, and that our life circumstances and demands create challenges and barriers outside of what this exercise addresses.

Evaluate each type of social connection you have using the following three categories:

- **Current obligation:** This is the amount of responsibility and effort you are putting into this type of relationship, ranked high, medium, or low.

- **Desired focus:** This is how much effort and energy you would *like* to be spending on a particular type of connection, ranked high, medium, or low.

- **Charge:** This is the total benefit and value of this relationship to you, expressed in a percentage. The maximum percentage you can have across all your relationships is 100.

Use this list of types of social connections to evaluate those applicable for you:

- Partner
- Children and in-laws
- Family of origin
- Personal relationships
- Work relationships
- Casual social connections
- Self

For instance, with your partner, you might currently be putting in a *medium* level of responsibility and effort—your current obligation. But you'd like to be putting in a *high* level of effort—your desired focus. Overall, your relationship with your partner gives you a 30 percent charge in your life.

As you review your results, notice differences between obligations and desires, as well as what is currently providing your social connections charge. Where are there gaps? I suggest you do this activity on a regular basis, as the closer you can get to a 100 percent charge with a balance of social connections, the better.

I personally have found this a wonderful way to demonstrate why a balance of social connections is important for our mental health, so we never put all our eggs in one basket. My partner said to me the other day, after sharing with me her relationship matrix, "Bill, I will always give you 100 percent of my 40 percent," meaning that her desire to our relationship was high, but that given her other social obligations, she only ever has 40 percent to give. This got me thinking about how many of us don't know where we get our social connections charge from, or how many of us are frustrated because we expect more from one relationship than the other has capacity to give because of their other relationship demands. For instance, if you are an introvert and require a lot of alone time to recharge (a social connection to self), you might have only 50 percent to give to others, and that 50 percent must be divided across work, romantic, and family relationships.

Your current circumstances and stage of life determine where you believe you need to focus your energy. For example, you might be caring for children or elderly parents. Finding balance can seem hard, but it is possible to take small steps daily to build your social connections charge in specific areas, such as discovering and building a new relationship or rekindling an old one. Regardless of your focus area, being successful at this requires attention, clarity on your desires, and management of your internal automatic negative thoughts and emotions.

As you begin your journey, one challenge with social connections is perspective. We can, for example, believe 98 percent of our relationships are fine. However, 2 percent may be in trouble. One strained critical relationship, like with a partner, can become overwhelming and result in us spending 98 percent of our effort to address the difficult 2 percent. This focus can, over time, lead to us distancing ourselves from all our other important relationships, which can increase feelings of isolation and risk of loneliness.

Let's talk about isolation and loneliness now, so we can then address ways to alleviate them.

2

Understand Isolation and Loneliness

ISOLATION AND LONELINESS can be measured by the degree to which a person feels emotionally disconnected from meaningful relationships with others. This disconnection is a state of mind that's influenced by both intrapersonal (i.e., how one feels and thinks about self) and interpersonal (i.e., how one interacts with others) relationships.[1]

Though isolation and loneliness are somewhat different, they are for the most part highly correlated. Just because someone feels isolated doesn't automatically mean they'll experience loneliness. One Angus Reid Institute poll reported nearly a quarter of Canadians experience extreme social isolation and loneliness.[2] Of those, there are:

- The desolate, who are both lonely and socially isolated (23 percent)
- The lonely but not isolated (10 percent)
- The isolated but not lonely (15 percent)

So, how is isolation a factor for you? It all depends on how you perceive isolation in your life. Here's a simple tool to help establish your perceived isolation load.

Perceived Isolation (PI) Load

Isolation factors are perceived barriers that consume your time, energy, and internal resources that contribute to social connections gaps. For each isolation factor listed here, indicate your average level of concern over the past 30 days on a scale from 1 (low) to 10 (high). Answer only those that apply to your current situation, and then add up your score to find your perceived isolation load.

- Financial challenges
- Family situation
- Stress level
- Fatigue
- Social network
- Parenting
- Mental health
- Addictive behaviours
- Work demand
- Elder care
- Self-confidence

- Abuse
- Inclusion
- Chronic illness
- Sexual orientation
- Gender bias
- Age discrimination
- Career satisfaction
- Education level
- Physical disability

Total score: ____

If your total score is between 20 and 60, your PI range is low; between 61 and 120 is moderate; and over 121 is high. The higher your score, the more barriers you perceive. Regardless of where you score, the purpose of this activity is to highlight barriers and to get you thinking about what is within your control to change. Life circumstances influence our day-to-day decisions. Some things we cannot change. But some things we can—when we are aware, accountable for what we can control, and motivated to act. I suggest you monitor this activity monthly as it can be highly correlated to loneliness. Often when we improve our resiliency and remove any mental barriers, we are well positioned to close social connections gaps. It is helpful to monitor your PI load and loneliness scores (see page 21) alongside your relationship matrix.

How Solitude Differs from Loneliness

It's important to not confuse loneliness with solitude. Solitude is when a person is alone but doesn't experience loneliness. Solitude is a peaceful state, whereas isolation and loneliness are emotionally painful states.

It can also be helpful to explore the differences between feeling lonely and loneliness. We've all felt lonely at moments in our life; there's no escaping this emotion. It's often temporary, but when feeling lonely becomes pervasive and chronic, it negatively impacts happiness and mental health. Feeling lonely for three days is not loneliness. Loneliness accumulates over time; how long varies. Typically, a few months is a strong trend of feeling lonely that can affect mood. People who experience loneliness often move one of two ways: 1) drive to move away from painful emotions by distraction, such as hiding in work, or 2) drive to protect, withdraw, and isolate to protect self from being hurt. A person who isolates from others can enter a state of seclusion, which often stems from loss of a loved one or a bad relationship.

The point is, a person can enjoy their time alone. However, such solitude is typically by choice, and often when the person feels ready to re-engage their social connections, they can do so effortlessly.

"Loneliness and the feeling of being unwanted is the most terrible poverty."

MOTHER TERESA

Loneliness Screen

Here's a quick screening test to determine the level of loneliness in your life. This tool is meant for educational purposes only—it's not a clinical assessment tool. On a typical day, how true are the below statements? Give yourself 0 for never, 1 for rarely, 2 for sometimes, or 3 for often.

- I often am unable to reach out and communicate with people around me.
- I often wish I had company, someone to talk to.
- I often feel that no one understands me.
- I often feel stressed about being alone.
- I often feel I'm waiting for people to call or write to me.
- I'm often sad because I end up doing things alone.
- I often find it hard to make friends.
- I often feel others are shutting me out.

Total score: ____

A total score of 1–8 is *low*. Most likely you're aware some days that you're lonely. Loneliness can be a hard thing to admit. The key to not falling into habits that lead to loneliness is to keep busy, don't isolate, and be open to the fact you may be pushing people away because of some internal fear of allowing them close to you. Pay attention and focus on activities that can increase your happiness.

A total score of 9–16 is *moderate*. At this level, you're aware that you're more alone than you want to be. Some try to rationalize that being alone is okay because they're an introvert. If this were truly okay, you would not be experiencing loneliness symptoms. Be aware for self-deception as an attempt to rationalize that loneliness is okay. Reading and learning about loneliness will assist in understanding what it is and how truly normal this feeling is. Many people feel alone; it's all too common. Understand that loneliness sneaks up on a person, and to change it requires awareness, actions, and some time to allow new relationships to form.

A total score of 17–24 is *high*. At this level, you likely feel trapped and alone and are struggling with loneliness. You don't need to be. The cure is to learn how to build meaningful and trusting relationships. Developing new habits and confidence can start to open new doors of opportunity. If you allow yourself to stay in this state for too long, you put yourself at risk of serious health issues. It's okay to act today and call your employee and family assistance program rep, doctor, or mental health professional to get support and make a plan.

Once you complete the above two tools, notice if there is a relationship between your isolation and loneliness scores. For example, if you have a low perceived isolation load, do you also have a low loneliness score? These are often aligned but not always. The difference can come down to resiliency, which allows you to push forward under adversity. We'll discuss the connection between loneliness and perceived isolation loads in more detail in chapter 5.

What's challenging for observers looking at another person is that both perceived isolation and loneliness are subjective. You may not be able to pick out an isolated and lonely person like you could one missing a limb. As with most mental health concerns, people experiencing isolation and loneliness often suffer in silence, and at different levels of intensity. Some who are highly functional and involved in the community hide it better than others who struggle more obviously.

Be careful of bias and stereotypes. Isolation and loneliness are much like alcoholism. Many people think alcoholics are living in skid row or on the street. This stereotype is wrong. The majority wake up and go to work every day. Many people experiencing isolation and loneliness do the same, while the absence of social connections in one or more parts of their life harms their mental health over time.

To make things even more complicated, there's no single, exact, universally accepted definition of these terms that fits every situation. It comes down to if a person thinks and feels they're isolated and lonely. It's a feeling, and feelings can be vague, messy, and unclear. The challenge with feelings is sometimes the person may feel a certain way and not connect the dots as to why. Without this insight, it's difficult to ever find happiness.

It's also helpful to understand that a person can feel isolated and lonely in different parts of their life. For example, Anne gets great value from her community-based volunteer work. However, with her family she feels unwelcome and not accepted, which leaves her feeling isolated and lonely. Compare Anne's situation with Gurpreet's. He has an amazing home life with children and a wife. But for him work is a challenge, as he doesn't feel psychologically safe there. His manager is difficult and at times a bully. His peers behave like his manager. Work is stressful, and Gurpreet doesn't feel he has any meaningful social connections at the office.

Isolation and loneliness can be situational. They don't have to impact every kind of relationship we have: family, partner, parent, work, community, and friendship. Each of us has a set of requirements (i.e., needs) for what we expect out of each type of relationship we enter. When these needs are not met and we perceive a gap, it can result in feeling not connected. Why this happens can vary from work schedule to emotional commitment to lack of psychological safety.

Take the example of going to work and not feeling psychologically safe with your team and manager. If you're not able to self-advocate, what typically happens is you experience avoidance, fear, and stress. But by developing your coping skills and resiliency, you can become more confident, calm, and able to articulate the boundaries you expect and what you'll tolerate.[3]

The phrase "moving away from isolation and loneliness" refers to fulfilling the specific social connections gaps that are missing. In the above work example, once psychological safety is achieved, fear is removed, and people who care are in place, the social connections gap will be closed.

Why you feel isolated and lonely may not be as important as what you learn to do with it. If you're open to becoming mindful, you'll be in a better position to self-evaluate whether you are experiencing common signs and symptoms of isolation and loneliness.

Emotional Loneliness

There are two forms of loneliness: emotional and social. Emotional loneliness refers to the absence of one-to-one relationships with individuals. Social loneliness is what happens when one person doesn't feel they fit or connect with a group or team.[4] In Part I, we'll focus primarily on emotional relationships. In Part III, we'll discuss the different kinds of authentic social relationships (e.g., home, work, partner, community).

Our emotions are typically a reaction to our current circumstances. We may feel isolated because of work demands, parenting, commuting, workload, or home chores. The day-to-day grind may be wearing us down; we feel trapped in a routine, and it seems like we have no time. The consequence is little to no time for social life, to engage in recreational activities, or to go out with our partner. Social connections gaps start to occur. Being in a marriage and having no time to connect can result in needs not being fulfilled.

When we feel strained, we may also feel anxious, depressed, or worried. These feelings can magnify our thoughts, which can influence our behaviours. How we cope with this pressure can vary from denial to engaging in feel-good behaviours to change our state, such as having an extra glass of wine with dinner—if we're not careful, that can go from one to four. Typically, our motivation is to feel better or to numb some perceived emotional pain, but if this feel-good behaviour is not monitored, it could lead to a substance use disorder, along with its own set of problems. I'm amazed at how many people end up addicted to a substance or behaviour (e.g., gambling) without seeing the signs that they're putting themselves in danger until they're in real trouble.

To understand isolation and loneliness, it's helpful to examine what people who have experienced them report. Here are common symptoms associated with feeling isolated and lonely:

- Feel empty, hollow inside, invisible, disappeared, unloved, resentful

- Feel disconnected from self

- Feel unworthy of or unable to have meaningful relationships

- Feel disconnected from others

- Suffer emotionally when thinking about social connections gaps

- Compensate for emotional discomfort through distractions, like hiding in work

- Avoid sharing true feelings with anyone
- Develop poor coping habits, such as overeating or using drugs or social media, to numb emotional pain
- Feel alone with no support
- Believe no one cares
- Worry there's no escape from these feelings
- Give up trying to fulfill social connections gaps (e.g., no longer seeks a partner)
- Regularly experience negative emotions (e.g., sadness)
- Often feel physically unwell (e.g., heart or stomach ailments)
- Avoid telling people how you feel due to stigma (e.g., shame)
- Feel one or more social connections are not aligned to wants, values, or purpose
- Unclear what to do to make things better

Check-in

Can you relate to any of the above symptoms? For each symptom you experience, rate how it applies to you on a scale of 1 (low impact on quality of life) to 5 (high impact). Sum them and get an average score.

The more symptoms you have and the higher your average score (e.g., 4), the more likely you are experiencing some degree of isolation and loneliness in one or more areas of your life.

Isolation and loneliness don't need to be a life sentence. With focus and commitment, many people have changed their circumstances; it's all about perspective and learning how to make change. Though self-awareness by itself is not a cure, it does create an opportunity to move from being on autopilot to being mindful as to what you're experiencing. When you can name feelings, you can challenge them. That's what we'll do in the next chapter, by examining what causes social connections gaps.

What Causes Social Connections Gaps?

WILLIAM GLASSER was a well-respected cognitive-behavioural psychiatrist with whom I had the privilege to take a cross-Canada tour to share his counselling theory called reality therapy. Throughout this five-city tour, I received some amazing mentoring from him on human behaviour. One of the key messages Glasser shared in almost every role-play he used to demonstrate reality therapy is that no matter what we do, think, or feel, we can never change our past. His message for all the counsellors and psychologists who wanted to be trained in his theory was that spending too much time and energy talking about a client's past increases the risk of getting lost in it. He insisted on focusing on what the person can change, what they think they want, what they really want, and what they're willing to do to get it.

A first step to move away from isolation and loneliness is to acknowledge that you really want to, and then create a mental picture of what your life will look like when you close your social connections gaps. As Glasser would say, your future starts *now*.

Of course, changing behaviour can be challenging, and simply knowing what you want and what success looks like is not enough. You must also be motivated and have a framework to act.

Barriers to Connection

The root cause of why you're struggling to develop meaningful social connections can vary. Attachment theory suggests that some people struggle to build healthy social connections because of inadequate early infant and childhood experiences where they lacked a sense of security or safety with at least one primary caregiver.[1] Some people are lonely because they were hurt in a past relationship or because someone special to them has died. Again, the reason may not be as crucial to curing isolation and loneliness as is developing self-awareness that there is an absence of social connections in some part of life.

Many lonely people know that if they could meet someone they trust to fulfill a social connections gap, they could feel better. Typically, there are different kinds of barriers, and we'll review these in more detail in Part II. The following is meant to introduce the concept of how thoughts can impact our experience. What we believe to be true shapes both our experiences and perceptions of our current reality.

Here are some common barriers that prevent a person from engaging in socially connective activities:

- Low self-confidence (i.e., the degree to which one likes one's self)

- Unrealistic expectations for self and others (e.g., perfection)

- Overreactive to unwanted challenges (e.g., tend to get angry and push people away, or "shut down" emotionally)

- Mental health concern (e.g., managing life stress is too challenging)
- Physical health issue
- Mobility issue
- Addictive disorder
- Moved to a new community, no current friends, not confident at networking
- Psychological safety issues at work
- Gaps in family support
- Social support systems gaps (e.g., friends, work, community)
- Lack of planned activities (e.g., hobbies, volunteering, sports, clubs, socializing with people regularly)
- Lack of time for a social life due to heavy work schedule (e.g., more than 60 hours per week)
- Lose many hours per week due to travel (e.g., flying or driving for work)

Check-in

Do you believe any of the above is a barrier that impacts your ability to engage in social connections activities?

On a scale of 1 (low risk) to 5 (high risk), rate the ones that you noted as a barrier.

Have you ever tried to remove any of the barriers you noted? If yes, what, if anything, helped?

Each barrier can impact your ability to close social connections gaps. Consider the person whose drive to get away from loneliness in a marriage results in their becoming a workaholic to keep their mind busy and distracted. When they go home and think about what's happening in their life, the pain of loneliness can be overwhelming. They've learned to get relief from loneliness by putting energy into their work. Or a lonely person can become angry or frustrated to the point of pushing people away, resulting in withdrawal.

Authentic connections are the goal, but a person can have many quality social connections and touchpoints that may not meet their needs. I believe that working toward closing social connections gaps is the first step and that those social connections become bonded and authentic over time. Now let's explore the role of technology in closing—or widening—social connections gaps.

4

The Connection Between Technology and Loneliness

WE USE TECHNOLOGY as a way to bridge the gap between ourselves and others, for personal, work, and educational reasons. But is technology actually capable of closing social connections gaps, thereby reducing isolation and loneliness?

The technology of smartphones and computers can be a wonderful way for people to stay connected. For the most part, these applications can assist people to feel socially connected and maintain social connections, which is different than looking to technology to fulfill social connections gaps. There are some healthy online social connections, and people have used technology to meet new people. However, I suspect that for new social connections to become authentic and lasting, the vast majority of people will need to meet in person to validate their online bond. Technology is a great facilitator, but it will never be the incubator that person-to-person interaction is for authentic human connections.

Having followers on social media feeds who provide lots of likes, or engaging in apps that allow for swiping left or right, seldom close social connections gaps, but they do fill a void, perhaps no different than having a glass of wine. The behaviour creates some perceived short-term benefit, but the root cause doesn't go away.

Getting to know someone in person is not the same as getting to know them online. Only when we truly get to know someone are we in a position to build a bond for honest, transparent, and meaningful social connection. I make this observation as it appears more people are looking for technology to close gaps that perhaps it cannot.

Just as we can't live without water, we can't live happily without social connections. I suspect that in the future our history books will tell stories about how society wasn't properly prepared to adapt to modern-day communications technology. I believe that the social connections that matter most are built and maintained as much as possible in person. The absence of in-person interaction can make it difficult for authentic connections to last.

Social Skills

When smart technology was introduced into society, I don't believe there was enough attention put on its negative consequences, such as addictive behaviours and loss of human interaction and communication skills. One of the biggest impacts I'm noticing is the erosion of human interaction skills, often called social skills. Many have lost the art of having authentic, in-person conversations; they'd rather text their feelings than talk about them.

We have a genetic need to interact with others. We're learning machines, but we need to be positioned to learn, such as by socially interacting. Building social skills is akin to a baby learning to walk. Babies are wired to learn this motor skill, but they don't learn how to take four steps in a row in a day. They learn from practice and from observing others. We learn how to build social connections by interacting with people.

One observation and concern I have about technology use in public and social interactions is how often a person you think you're talking to is not present; they're focused on their device. How many times have you been talking with someone who got a text and stopped talking to you to check it? How often do you drop over to visit someone without texting, calling, or emailing first that you're coming? It appears to me we are losing the ability to just be humans and connect naturally.

The good news is I'm noticing more people who want to get back to basics and are turning technology off at night, unplugging, engaging in community activities, going on hikes, and visiting people they care about. Humans need humans! Also, I believe that unplugging can help people reduce their risk of burnout.[1]

Another troublesome observation I have about technology is that some people sit hyper-focused for hours waiting for a single response to a text. While waiting, they may not be aware that an automatic negative thought like "They don't care about me" may bubble up, when in actuality the recipient may not even have read the text yet.

With the instant world of communications come many advantages as well as expectations. When these expectations are not discussed or agreed upon, no matter the kind of relationship, it's common for a person to feel rejected or slighted if someone doesn't return their text or email. Why did they not just pick up the phone and call? Perhaps because they may have lost that skill and the confidence to make a call. I recall asking my son, "Did you know it's okay to just call someone without texting them to tell them you're about to call them?" His response: "Dad, no one does that." Wow, I know I'm getting older and remember the rotary phone, but really?

Another challenge with technology is what I call false social connections: for example, you're connected to someone on LinkedIn that you don't know and will never take the time to get to know. Social connections must be meaningful to have a positive effect on your mental health, and for them to be meaningful, you need to communicate and get to know each other. To even get to this point, both parties must be open to picking up a phone and talking—then perhaps meeting for tea. This creates an opportunity to move this false social connection to an authentic social connection. For any relationship to evolve to an authentic connection requires two-way commitment, communication, and focus. Building authentic connections takes time, energy, and some risk, as not all relationships work out. Oh, and yes, they involve face-to-face interaction. Have I mentioned that yet?

When it comes to technology, I've also observed people overestimating the value online relationships have compared to in-person relationships. I call it the loneliness paradox, which is when a person has 500 false social connections online that they interact with at different levels of frequency. However, if the person ended up sick in the hospital, they would not be surprised if none of those 500 showed up to visit them. Inside they know they have no real social connections; they have a bunch of online acquaintances. The paradox is the more time and energy a person spends on social media and gaming, the less time and energy they have to make in-person social connections, which are the ones that will show up in times of need.

I've observed first-hand two of my children involved in social media and gaming communities, where it appears they have thousands of connections, but as their parent I know they're often feeling isolated and lonely. Why? Because they're not focused on closing their social connections gaps. They're spending their time doing what I call "surface touch technology interactions."

Technology has a place to help us humans be connected, but it will never be able to fill the role of authentic social connections. "People need to be able to touch people to love them," I said once during a talk. I'm not 100 percent sure this statement is true, but it sounded good at the time, and a lot of people nodded in agreement. In partner relationships, you need to be able to touch the other person to be socially connected. Distance partner relationships are okay, but without an opportunity for intimacy and sex, they're likely going to fail if at least one person yearns to touch. Research shows that couples who are able to engage in physical contact like sex not only benefitted from its physiological benefits but also strengthened a more positive social connection with their partners.[2] Even in non-intimate relationships, I've experienced first-hand that chatting on the phone with my football buddies is not remotely the same as interacting with them in person and feeling their energy.

One problem gaining more traction and focus is the risk of addictive compulsive behaviour such as internet addiction and gaming. Like any addiction, compulsive internet use can end up pushing people away. Social media and gaming addiction disorders can operate similarly to pathological gambling, where the stimulus and rush gained by getting a comment or like is rewarding and fuels the drive and obsession to get such perceived awards that never have any lasting effect or benefit. While smartphone technology is promoted and sold for all its benefits, seldom do I see or hear a warning about its addictive qualities. Cigarettes were once thought to be harmless, too.

Today, young people are having to go to detox to get off their technology, as they've become addicted to it.[3]

Over time, this compulsive behaviour can result in gaps in social connections. The habit of being online for hours a day creates a barrier to engaging in social interactions with others in person, and their world becomes smaller.

I don't want to make technology out as the enemy of happiness. It's a facilitator and also a risk to eroding and losing social skills if not used appropriately. Because technology is easy to use, requiring less effort than talking on the phone or visiting in person, my concern is too many are not aware of the unintended consequences of their micro-decisions regarding how they interact. As a society, we have failed to educate people on how misuse and overuse of technology can negatively impact social connections and become a contributing factor to isolation and loneliness.

> **Check-in**
>
> Do you think smartphone technology has helped or hurt the average person in building meaningful social connections? List the pros and cons of smartphone technology in closing social connections gaps.
>
> Do you believe that smartphone technology has had any negative impact on your social skills? If yes, be specific.

When a person experiences gaps in social connections in one or more areas of their life over an extended period, they can feel loneliness. Isolation and loneliness are personal; no two people have the same experience. The degree to which you experience isolation and loneliness is dependent on the perceived severity of your social connections gaps, number of barriers, and how long you've been experiencing feelings of isolation and loneliness. Moving away from isolation and loneliness begins with being able to name them. The next step is being open to learning how to escape the mental trap.

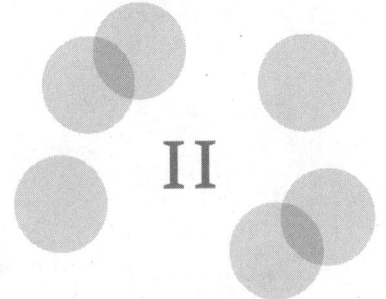

Escaping the Mental Trap

How Mental Traps Form

How does a mental trap form? Once the mind accepts one random negative thought as true, it leads to self-doubt and the negative feelings associated with it. These feelings shape mood. The mental trap creates internal rules and limitations that impact decision making, taking over like a weed that impacts both the unconscious and conscious mind. The stronger the trap, the more restrictive it becomes, and the less positive the person's outlook.

A mental trap inhibits self-confidence and drains energy, which can prevent a person from enjoying life, taking chances, trying something different, speaking their mind, meeting people, travelling, joining clubs, enjoying a social activity, or quitting a bad job out of fear they may not be good enough to find a better one. When not managed, a mental trap will stop a person from learning how to close their social connections gaps. By learning how to unlock your mental trap, you can create positive thinking, emotions, and expectations that will allow you to close social connections gaps.

This chapter will explore four factors that when not confronted or managed can contribute to the development of a mental trap that can impact your behaviour, thinking, expectations, and emotions. These factors are: 1) perceived isolation, 2) the fight or flight response, 3) thoughts, and 4) negative emotions. By exploring these factors, you'll become more aware about how mental traps are formed, providing you with a foundation to learn how to stop judging yourself.

The Long-Term Effects of the Mental Trap

Pain, pleasure, and fear motivate most human behaviours. These can be influenced by both our unconscious and conscious mind. The unconscious mind doesn't need to be taught how to be fearful, nor does it need to be taught how to feel pain or enjoy pleasure. We're hardwired to experience these feelings. However, our mental health is directly impacted by how we learn to manage pain, pleasure, and fear.

Feeling trapped in isolation and loneliness isn't necessary; you can learn how to unlock your mental trap. I want to anchor the point that for the context of this book, the purpose of unlocking the mental trap is to close social connections gaps. However, you can use the micro-skills taught in the resiliency and cognitive-behavioural approach (CBA) chapters to help you move past other perceived barriers such as job loss or lack of money.

The longer your mental trap impacts your thinking and emotions, the greater the risk that you'll get stuck in it and lose hope. With little to no hope, it's common to believe you have no choice or control of your current life situation. Your mental trap, when locked and filled with negative thinking and emotions, is how you'll perceive your reality, regardless if the thoughts are true.

Unfortunately, some people stay stuck in their mental trap for days, weeks, and even years. Before you can achieve your full potential for making new social connections and building authentic connections, you must learn to unlock your mental trap. You must understand that your thinking and emotions are holding you back from seeing how you can move forward.

Not until you believe there are things you can do to unlock your mental trap will anything change. All I ask is for you to be open to the possibility that you can learn how to see the world differently than you do now.

> **Check-in**
>
> On a scale of 1 (no impact) to 10 (high impact), how much has a feeling of fear and pain (e.g., rejection) impacted your ability to close social connections gaps? Anything greater than a 3 is likely higher than you want.
>
> On a scale of 1 (low) to 10 (high), how much hope do you have that you can close the social connections gaps you have in your life?

Whatever your score, add the ideas of this book to your daily routine for at least 60 days, and you may find your perspective changes. The longer you walk down this path and just try, the more likely you'll learn new habits so they become as routine as brushing your teeth or getting dressed. Putting the effort in will help you learn about yourself, which in turn will help you determine if you can do this alone or if you would benefit from additional support.

> **Stay safe**
>
> At any point, if you start to become overwhelmed and believe you need help, call your employee and family assistance representative, 911, local crisis line, or mental health line.

When stuck in a mental trap, it's normal to feel overwhelmed by emotional pain (e.g., fear, regret, worry, sadness, or anxiety). The severity of the mental trap you experience will be determined by the degree of your emotional pain, the level of negative internal dialogue you're having about your future, and how much hope you have that things can get better.

Four Factors That Contribute to Building Mental Traps

I suspect you've had days when things seemed easier, and life and work were not as difficult. The thoughts we have about ourselves and others position us to be open or closed to interacting with others. It's difficult to have meaningful social connections with others if we don't have them with ourselves. Unlocking your mental trap can help you learn to have more self-compassion and to give yourself a break. Self-compassion is when you can understand, accept, and love yourself.[1] It's not about self-esteem. It's about self-acceptance even when you fail; it's about being mindful that you don't need to be perfect; it's about not needing to prove yourself to others; it's about accepting that you're worthy and deserving of love from yourself and others.

Self-awareness theory teaches that we're not our thoughts, but an observer who's observing our thoughts.[2] It's helpful to understand that the thinker (you) is separate from your thoughts. This theory explains that human beings, for the most part, compare themselves against two perceived standards:

Pass: You find acceptance and alignment with the standard set for self and outcome. For example, "I'm in a loving and caring relationship"; "I have loving and caring friends."

Fail: You find some discrepancy between what you want and what you have. For example, "I'm not satisfied in this marriage; it's not meeting my emotional needs"; "I don't trust the people I work with."

Mental traps don't allow much room in the middle, for a grey zone with elements of both passing and failing: "I love my job but I wish I were working on the leadership team rather than as a field rep." The mental trap can be challenging if we're not aware when we're stuck in failure. When we don't think we can change something to our favour, it's common to avoid trying. This attitude contrasts with having hope and the belief that things can get better if we're committed to learning and taking a chance. How you navigate each of these four factors plays a role in what you allow yourself to think is possible.

Factor 1: Perceived Isolation

How intense a mental trap becomes will depend on the frequency, duration, and intensity (FDI) of unwanted thoughts

"A trap is only a trap if you don't know about it. If you know about it, it's a challenge."

CHINA MIÉVILLE

and emotions that limit your confidence to close your social connections gaps. The greater the FDI, the greater the risk that the mental trap will lead to behaviours that contribute to feelings of isolation and loneliness.

Take another look at your perceived isolation load from the assessment exercise on page 18. The more perceived barriers there are, the higher the likelihood some social connections gaps will exist. The combination of perceived barriers and FDI can predict the likelihood your mental health is being strained due to gaps in your social connections. The degree of hope you have that you can improve your situation is important. When you have no hope to close social connections gaps, you're less likely to see a path to building meaningful connections. This is one sign that your mental trap is hurting your belief system.

Perceived isolation barriers—covert or overt—if not dealt with can impact your ability to fulfill social connections and lead to feelings of loneliness.

Consider this covert example. If you commute four hours and work an average of nine hours each day, by the time you get home and do some basic chores, you have no energy to interact. However, you may have a caring, patient partner with whom you're bonded, so you don't feel lonely. But you do feel isolated from being able to engage in activities you like, such as playing your sport of choice. This isolation can result in yearning and missing the social connections you had when you played sports.

An overt example is being in a marriage where you feel trapped, unhappy, and are experiencing loneliness.

Loneliness expert John Cacioppo found that perceived isolation (how a person sees their world) is much more powerful than objective isolation (how their world is).[3] I was caught by the notion of how perceived isolation—whether good or bad—in the absence of meaningful social connections can predict loneliness.

Before my dad passed away, he was trapped in his bed. Due to neurological damage, his muscles weren't allowing him to function. He couldn't get out of bed and was objectively isolated. There was no perception here; it was his reality. However, because he had his family and caring nurses around him, he claimed he never felt alone. I know, because I asked him, and he said his days went by just fine, and he didn't feel alone. He missed his freedom but accepted his circumstances. He openly talked about the importance of social connections for his happiness at the end of his life and how they had a positive impact on his mental health.

Perceived isolation is what one believes to be true; two people in the same situation can have two different perceptions of it. For example, Fred perceives he doesn't have enough money to go out, so he feels trapped and stays home alone. However, Jim, who is in the same financial boat, goes for a walk with a friend and says hello to people as they stroll. The fact is, you don't need money to build or maintain social connections. Facts and perception are two different realities. When a person perceives something is holding them back, they can create an internal belief that defines their reality.

Perceived isolation can be difficult to notice or detect because you can get used to your reality and accept it as normal. The longer you live with some perceived isolation factor(s) that you believe is preventing you from engaging in social connections, the bigger your social connections gaps can become.

Perceived isolation is seldom unidimensional—just one factor. Here's an example of perceived isolation that's multi-dimensional. Jane went to work daily feeling isolated because of several factors: her age, gender, job satisfaction, and financial health. She believed she could never find another job because of her age and being a female in a male-dominated industry. She lost her joy for work and stayed because of her debts. Jane's perceived isolation load became the barrier and reason for why she spent more time alone after work. To cope, she created a routine of online shopping at night, which resulted in driving up her credit card debt.

> **Check-in**
>
> Leveraging the perceived isolation research, I designed a short survey that I put online with the *Globe and Mail*. You can take the Perceived Isolation-Loneliness Effect survey on the Howatt HR website.[4]
>
> Print out your survey results to keep as a frame of reference for what your perceived barriers can be. The survey can also provide insight into the link between perceived isolation and loneliness.

As you review each of the perceived isolation barriers, reflect on how you think they could be an obstacle in your life and evaluate your degree of concern on a scale of 1 (no concern) to 10 (major concern):

- **Financial:** you feel restricted because of money challenges
- **Work demand:** your workload feels overwhelming and takes over your life
- **Bullying:** you don't feel psychologically safe in your workplace or another environment

- **Job satisfaction:** you feel stuck in a job you don't like
- **Gender:** you believe your gender identity is restricting your career or other opportunities
- **Mental illness:** your concern about stigma makes you reluctant to discuss your mental health with anyone
- **Return to work:** you felt isolated and alone while off work and now worry about how you'll be perceived when you return
- **Manager-employee relationship:** you don't feel confident about your relationship with your manager and feel isolated and unsure about job security
- **Team:** you're not sure why but you don't feel like you're fitting in; you feel excluded from your team, group, or community

Becoming aware of your perceived isolation barriers lets you objectively evaluate their impact. We live in a fast-paced world, and most of us have routines and daily habits that we're not paying close attention to. Consider how often you wake up and begin your day on autopilot. You follow a routine to get ready for work, without realizing many decisions have already been made. This routine can fuel your mental trap if you're not aware of how your daily choices result in not putting enough focus on fulfilling social connections gaps or maintaining social connections. That you have choices and don't have to be trapped is a helpful insight to begin thinking about how to remove your barriers.

William Glasser, the author of reality therapy, taught that we all have four basic, conscious genetic needs: love and belonging, power, freedom, and fun.[5] The most important is love and belonging. One way to stress-test this theory is to imagine you only had 72 hours to live. Would you trade all your money and status to spend those last few days with the people you value and love? There's nothing more important than social connections for mental health and happiness, and keeping aware of that truth can motivate you to learn how to close social connections gaps. The fact is, we're genetically wired to crave social connections.

Glasser taught that to obtain our wants, we must be clear on what they are and what they look like. He called these "quality world pictures." Mental traps can dampen our clarity of what we want. Glasser often asked people what they don't want (e.g., to be alone), followed by what they do want (e.g., to have a caring friend they trust). He would then ask them what they think they can do to get what they want. The power of this question is that it implies that the person has agency to obtain what they want. Once they see what they want, they can begin the journey to achieve it.

Mental traps don't typically form overnight but over a period of time. There can be different root causes, from a perceived barrier to a loss of an important personal relationship due to conflict, divorce, or death. Loss of a valued social connection—like a work partnership, family member, or marriage—can be traumatic and result in grieving, withdrawing, and socially isolating. Regardless of the root cause of the barrier or loss, if not addressed it can lead to negative feelings, thoughts, and behaviours. How we react or learn to cope defines how greatly it strengthens the hold our mental trap has on our perception of hope.

Less effective coping can lead to an isolation and loneliness feedback loop. Effective coping can support your mental health. Less effective coping strategies, such as withdrawing and not interacting with others, may appear to be helpful for self-protection at first. But when this strategy is used over an extended period, you're at increased risk of isolating yourself from others, which can increase the risk of loneliness, or at the very least disrupt your ability to fulfill basic social connections.

> **Check-in**
>
> - Is your mental trap a barrier to closing social connections gaps?
> - Are you motivated to loosen your mental trap?
> - Do you believe that if you changed your negative thinking, it would help you unlock your mental trap?

Consider this scenario that illustrates how negative thinking and less effective coping strategies can snowball. Amita is 44 and a single mom who must work all day to make enough money to pay her bills. Her husband died a few years ago from cancer. She has the daily responsibility of taking care of her seven-year-old daughter and her 83-year-old mother. Amita is an only child; her dad passed away, leaving her mother with no partner and no day-to-day support. No other family members live in the area. Amita is the only family member available to support her mother. She also knows her mother has no financial resources to hire anyone to help.

Amita cares for and loves her mom and daughter deeply. She's often tired at the end of her day and feels overwhelmed keeping up with the demands of home and work. Most days, she wakes up happy to support her daughter and mother, although a few days each month she feels a sense of loneliness before going to bed. She misses having companionship. From time to time she wonders what it would be like to start dating. However, after a few minutes, she dismisses that thought as not a remote possibility. Why? Her mental trap fires off a negative train of thoughts: "Forget about it; I'm going to be alone until Mom and Nupur don't need me. This is just how it has to be."

The day-to-day grind is slowly taking a toll on Amita's mental health and happiness. She constantly feels under stress with no idea how to improve her situation or to create an opportunity for herself. Between work and taking care of her daughter and mother, she has no time or energy left. She uses food to cope with stress and to feel better. Her mental trap tricks her into believing that eating at night when she's not hungry is okay. Her new habit has resulted in her putting on 25 pounds. Now Amita, who used to take pride in her appearance, is not happy with the extra weight, and that's adding another reason why she believes it will be hard to find someone, as she doesn't like the way she looks.

If Amita's mental trap is locked and she continues to experience her perceived isolation barriers (responsibility to take care of her daughter and mom), her risk of loneliness will increase. If Amita had the confidence and clarity, she could start dating again. But not until she learns how to overcome her negative self-talk will she try or be open to trying. She may be missing opportunities that are being presented to her because of her mindset.

> **Check-in**
>
> - Can you relate to why Amita will remain trapped if she doesn't have the resources to challenge her negative thoughts?
> - What was one key observation you took from learning more about perceived isolation?
> - Do you believe perceived isolation barriers contribute to your mental trap?
> - Are you now more aware of your perceived isolation barriers?

Factor 2: The Fight or Flight Response

The rational, conscious brain is what helps us solve and deal with life problems in an objective way. It can process information quickly, find relevant facts, and make thoughtful decisions. However, when it's not sure what to do and feels overwhelmed, this leaves an opening for the unconscious brain to turn on.

The unconscious (caveman) brain exists to protect us from danger and help ensure our survival. Keeping us safe and alive is its core function, and it does that well: we're at the top of the food chain. However, when our caveman brain turns on when it's not needed to keep us safe from lethal danger, it can create unnecessary anxiety, worry, and fear.

Even with all our modern advancements, our fight or flight survival response system hasn't evolved. When it turns on, it's at 100 percent, whether a sabre-toothed tiger is chasing us or someone has just cut us off in traffic. When our unconscious brain perceives danger, it turns on. A person who engages in road rage is likely unaware that they've been emotionally hijacked. In this state, cognitive ability is diminished, and emotions like rage stem from fear.

The fight or flight response is the same for both lethal and non-lethal situations, and if you're not aware of how it operates, it can be both frightening and confusing when it turns on. In the example of road rage, it can result in acting out or other "fight" behaviours that often don't improve the situation.

The fight or flight response system operates 24/7, constantly looking to protect you from danger. There's no off switch. Its response is not concerned about the future; its only concern is to protect you at the moment. The fight or flight response system still has a purpose and is extremely helpful. Consider when you're driving your car. You're not likely to be hyper-focused or worried about getting killed in an accident. Though you must be alert and pay attention, you're fortunate that your fight or flight response system is on. Why? It acts as your unconscious, automatic defence reflex, doing its best to detect danger and react before you're aware of it. Think about a time someone cut you off, and recall how without thinking your foot automatically hit the brakes before your conscious mind knew what was going on. This reflex is hardwired; you don't have to think about it.

Because the fight or flight response in the unconscious brain is hardwired, it can override your conscious brain. The shot of fear you experience after you've been cut off is meant to teach you to avoid this kind of situation in the future. Think about a caveman wading into a body of water and getting bitten by some larger creature. His experience and fear response would caution him against doing the same thing again, to suffer the same fate. Fear is a protector and meant to be a teacher.

The problem with fear is that it's not rational. Your conscious brain must process the event that has just happened and put it into perspective. Fear is necessary for survival and self-protection; however, you can learn how to not allow irrational fear to control you. Irrational fear is being afraid of something that's not lethal, such as engaging in a conversation with a stranger. You may fear you will be rejected or judged, but, provided you're in a safe place, there's little risk you'll be hurt physically.

When not managed, fear can control your behaviour. It can strengthen your mental trap and add to feelings of isolation. For example, if you're fearful of being rejected and don't engage in social activities, you increase your risk of feeling isolated and lonely.

The fight or flight system response has a third choice, which is typically called freeze. In some circumstances, our brain can become almost short-circuited by fear, and we just freeze. This reaction is not helpful, because it keeps us in a state of fear that neither protects us nor moves us away from danger.

Here's an example of how the fight or flight system can produce self-protective responses. Joe is a middle manager whose boss is sexually harassing him. Joe is embarrassed and not sure how to deal with this situation. He fears that if he reports his situation to human resources, they'll laugh at him, do nothing, or, even worse, his boss will find out and fire him. Joe's working in a psychologically unsafe workplace, feeling socially isolated, alone, and fearful. His concern about psychological safety is an example of a perceived isolation barrier.

Joe's boss has become more aggressive and intentional with her sexual harassment. She had just been making verbal comments, but one day while Joe was bending over to get something out of his desk, she grabbed his butt. Joe's fight or flight response automatically turned on and he jumped out of the way quickly. Once he turned around and realized what his boss had done, he froze. He was lost for words and overwhelmed cognitively, emotionally, and physiologically. The experience could make him feel powerless, feed his mental trap, and make his situation even more difficult.

> **Check-in**
>
> Have you been trained on how to manage your fight or flight response in a way that doesn't cause you or others emotional strain?
>
> If no, you're not alone. Most of us have never been taught how the fight or flight response system works. By increasing your awareness of the fight or flight response, you'll better understand how fear can inhibit behaviours that may actually be what you want.
>
> Can you picture any situation in the past month where your fight or flight response fired off in a non-lethal situation?
>
> How did you cope? Did your coping actions help or hurt?

Factor 3: Thoughts

You don't need to be a neuroscientist to understand that your thinking plays a major role in influencing what you do. Your mental health is dependent on how well you can manage the interactions between your thoughts, feelings, and physiology (e.g., fear response).

During stressful periods when your fight or flight response has been activated or you think about something that brings up fear, how you regulate your arousal level affects how you perceive the world. Thinking you have no control over your world contributes to building your mental trap.

Another way thinking affects our perception of the world lies in what we think we want. Miswanting is the act of being wrong about what and how much we would like something.[6] It refers to the notion that getting more of something will make us happier. For example, "If only I could win $1 million, I'd be happier." But research has found that lottery winners after one year are no happier than someone who has experienced a serious accident (e.g., loss of a limb).[7] It's a problem many are not aware of.

Thinking that attaining more of something will make us happy, as well as perceiving a difference between what we want and expect, can result in unnecessary stress. Stuff doesn't make us happy; what we think of ourselves and the quality of our social connections make us happy. Focusing energy on money, status, or career goals can lead to isolation and loneliness if we don't learn to slow down and enjoy what we have. Miswanting can become a barrier that can lead to feeling isolated. For example, becoming a billionaire but having no one to share your wealth with may not feel like a wonderful experience. I know some very wealthy people who aren't happy, and I'm not sure they'll become happy until they can learn to be comfortable with who they are and not push people away.

It can be difficult to deal with a mental trap if you're not aware of how your beliefs and wants drive your behaviour. Consider these three strategies as to how a person may cope with social connections gaps:

- They shut down and no longer try.

- They engage in behaviours (e.g., overusing alcohol) to numb feelings of loneliness.

- They put all their attention into their work to escape feelings of loneliness. What can be confusing to onlookers is this person can appear productive—excelling in work, volunteering, or parenting. However, a social connections gap, like lack of a partner relationship, acts like a toothache. Whenever they slow down or stop, the pain intensifies, so to escape it they speed up again.

One challenge with mental traps is we humans get used to things. Immune neglect is our tendency to adapt and cope with negative events. Daniel Gilbert, in *Stumbling on Happiness*, explains that it's common to think about one event and forget another that happened to us. We tend to get used to our current situation. Gilbert suggests that one shortcoming of our imagination is we too often buy into the limited thinking it provides as possible options to life problems, which is not that imaginative.[8] We might only imagine our future will be the same as our experience today. This limits our belief in our potential to close social connections gaps and strengthens the mental trap.

But research has found that what we predict in a negative state is usually not accurate; it's not what happens in real life. For example, a person who's upset and says, "I'll never meet another person who'll like me," is likely wrong. Making this statement isn't an accurate prediction. If they focus on self-care and building social connections, they're apt to meet someone who likes them. The takeaway is just because you don't see a brighter future today doesn't mean it's not possible. Just because you don't see a possibility or answer, that doesn't mean it doesn't exist.

While studying for one of my degrees I heard one line—I can't recall who said it—that has stuck with me for the past 30 years: "What we think, we become." Choice theory author Glasser taught that every human being with a functional, healthy brain has total control of their behaviours, some control over their thinking, and little to no control over their feelings.[9] However, because our behaviours, thinking, feelings, and physiology are all connected, where thinking goes feelings follow.

Glasser used the metaphor of a front-wheel-drive car. On the front wheels are thoughts and behaviours, and on the back wheels are physiology (fight or flight) and emotions (mood). This suggests that where the front wheels go, the rear wheels have no choice but to follow. Some people, though, appear to be in a rear-wheel-drive car, based on how they underreact or overreact emotionally. It's evident they're struggling with their mood and not controlling their fight or flight responses in non-lethal situations. However, Glasser purported that once they become consciously aware, take accountability for their choices, and learn and accept how to drive their front-wheel-drive car, they can take control of their life choices. Awareness is the first step to learning how to take control of one's behaviour system.

Choice theory insists that we all have choice. However, this can be difficult to grasp when we're caught in emotions and feel we have no choice. Whenever we experience a difference between what we want and what we have, choice theory refers to this as pure pain. This pain will continue until the situation is resolved or distracted. With pain related to isolation and loneliness, this is where less effective coping behaviours can happen. They may include avoiding people so you don't get hurt, engaging in addictive behaviours, and being consumed by work so you don't think about your social connections gaps. Some people appear to be happy and productive and are experiencing loneliness. Sometimes they're simply not aware of what's happening or why they feel the way they do, and they can develop another problem, like anxiety or work addiction. The root cause of their stress is a social connections gap. I've seen this scenario play out a few times in counselling. The position we typically took was improving a relationship gap as a strategy to support the treatment of anxiety or other mental illness, including addiction.

Regardless of such less effective coping behaviours, until the social connections gap is closed, this pure pain will never go away. It's common for the intensity of the pain to vary, based on which less effective coping behaviours are in play.

If you're caught in negative emotions, your negative thinking is a root cause. One key to breaking out of your mental trap is to become aware and notice how your thinking influences your feelings. Negative thinking often is rooted in faulty thinking, which is when your unconscious brain fires off one or more automatic thoughts that you accept as being true. These negative thoughts come out of some perceived fear or faulty logic that's not grounded in facts.

During my keynotes, I often ask the following question to get the participants' responses: "Why does the single guy in the bar who's interested in the single woman he noticed not get up to introduce himself?" The typical response is because he's fearful of rejection.

I nod and then ask my next question: "Two plus two equals?" There's often a pause, and then I have to say I'm not trying to trick them and ask the question again. Once I get the right answer, I go on to explain why I asked this math question. It provides an example of how cognitive schemas work.

Cognitive schemas are the set of filters that define how we think others see us, as well as how we view the world and how we evaluate success. Negative cognitive schemas act like spyware in a computer: they run in the background without anyone knowing about them. We don't need to think about what two plus two equals; we know the answer is four.

In the case of the guy in the bar, he sees the woman and does his math equation when he thinks about getting up and introducing himself. Why he doesn't get up is because his negative cognitive schema filter analyzed his chances of a positive response from her as zero. His automatic decision was it was safer to not try, so there is no risk of being rejected because that's what would likely happen.

Aaron Beck, one of the founders of the modern-day cognitive-behavioural approach, suggested that cognitive schemas influence our beliefs and assumptions about the world.[10] The problem with negative cognitive schemas is they can be formed on faulty assumptions, which simply aren't true. However, when we believe they're true, they can paralyze us from trying, which strengthens the mental trap.

Based on your life experience, you likely have developed some negative cognitive schemas that have contributed to your mental trap. Why cognitive schemas are so powerful in controlling behaviour is they're automatic. And because they're automatic, we don't debate them; we believe they're true.

> **Check-in**
>
> - Be sad for 30 seconds.
> - Be happy for 30 seconds.
> - Picture yourself in your favourite spot for 30 seconds.
> - Now raise your right arm.
> - Which of the four tasks was the easiest for you to do? Interestingly, many pick one of the two emotions over the visualizing and arm movement. If you probe a bit to discover how they created the emotion, they will share that they thought of a particular situation. The insight from this exercise is that thoughts come before feelings.

It's helpful to become aware of how automatic thoughts can drive feelings and mood. When they're not managed, cognitive schemas can prevent you from pursuing what you want, like the guy in the bar whose cognitive schema triggered fear of failing and stopped him from trying. The consequence is the guy will never know the woman, who could have become a valuable social connection.

When you're unsure how to challenge your automatic negative thoughts, your mental trap can take a stronger hold of your behaviours. The guy's automatic thoughts stopped him from trying. What was the worst case for him? What was the best case? What's certain is that by not trying he'll never know the best case.

Negative cognitive schemas come from faulty self-talk based on our experiences with the world. If not challenged over time, faulty self-talk harms our self-worth. There are different kinds of faulty self-talk, such as:

- Faulty logic (e.g., believing you are unworthy of love)
- Learned helplessness (e.g., believing there's no opportunity to improve a situation)
- Negative self-perceptions (e.g., "I'm a difficult person to love") that result in self-programming
- Catastrophizing, or overestimating the meaning of an action (e.g., not returning your text means the person doesn't care)

Faulty thinking trains the unconscious brain to develop negative cognitive schemas that bias how we see and interact with the world. Russ Harris explains in his book *ACT Made Simple* that cognitive fusion means our thoughts drive our behaviour.[11] The risk is that we accept our negative thoughts as absolute truth.

Factor 4: Negative Emotions

Emotions when not managed influence our thinking and our perceptions of what's possible. During our waking hours on any typical day, the range of emotions we experience can be vast, from happiness to anger, sadness, frustration, concern, and love. Emotions provide the spice and flavour to our daily experiences, which can be perceived as good or bad. For the most part, emotions move us either toward people or away. Shame and guilt can move us away, while love and joy can move us toward people.

Our mood is influenced by the dominance and frequency of the kinds of emotions we're experiencing. The longer we experience worry, the more likely our mood will be anxious. And the longer we experience feelings and thoughts that drive self-doubt, the more likely our mood will become depressed.

Emotions are experienced at different levels of intensity. When we're having a wonderful time with lots of fun and belly laughter to the point of tears, there's no question what emotion we're experiencing: happiness. Compare that to when we're feeling down or just "off."

> **Check-in**
>
> Estimate what percentage of the day you experience positive emotions.
>
> Estimate what percentage of the day you experience negative emotions.
>
> How would you describe your mood over the last two weeks?
>
> One way to define mental health is your level of satisfaction with your current station in life. Mental health is experienced through feelings. When you don't feel good, it impacts your desire and motivation. To make any change it's important to be motivated, to want to change, and to be willing to act.[12] Thinking about change isn't the same as being open to learning how to change. Changing feelings often first requires learning how to change negative thinking.

Monitoring Your Emotions

When you're not aware of your emotions or what emotions you spend most of your day feeling, you have little ability to evaluate or change them. One step to unlocking your mental trap is to become aware of the role emotions play in strengthening its hold on your mood. Many people don't measure and monitor their daily emotions, which is a missed opportunity for self-correcting. I highly recommend daily mood monitoring to become conscious of your mood trends, so you can intervene early if you notice a downswing.

The broaden-and-build theory teaches that our experience of three key positive emotions affects how we see the world:[13]

- **Joy** focuses us on embracing positive thoughts and actions that build up our intelligence and physical and social resources

- **Contentment** helps to put our views of the world and self in perspective

- **Interest and curiosity** promote the drive to seek new knowledge to experience and try different things that spark personal growth

The degree to which you experience each of these positive emotions daily can predict your mood, mental health, and longevity. Happier people typically live longer lives, with less risk of physical and mental illness.

The broaden-and-build theory also suggests there are three negative emotions that can wear down our mental health: depression, disappointment, and indifference. The frequency, duration, and intensity (FDI) of these emotions predict mood.

These negative emotions can explain why some people shut down and don't try, because their mood is so down, and hope is low. When negative emotions become a habit, some people may not try to maintain their social connections because they don't have any energy. Negative moods are draining and isolating. The result is greater absence of social connections, which only increases the risk of experiencing loneliness and fuels more negative emotions.

Feelings of loneliness can result in increased feelings of disappointment and depression that can reinforce the mental trap, suggesting that it's safer to avoid people. The combination of negative emotions and negative self-talk ("Why would anyone want to be with me? I'm not loveable") can result in feeling even more locked in a mental trap and can become a stronger barrier to trying to fill a social connections gap.

EACH OF these four factors influences the development of mental traps and how strongly such traps determine how we view and interact with the world. What stops many of us from getting the kinds of social connections we crave is not the external world; it's the battle we have with our internal world. Our mental traps impact our mental health and affect how confident we are. Unlocking our mental traps allows us to develop a kind relationship with ourselves and to be open to closing social connections gaps.

This chapter provided some insights into the factors that will help you move away from unhelpful thoughts and feelings. The purpose of this preparation work is to put yourself in the best position to build or repair social connections, which we'll discuss in future chapters on forming authentic connections.

How to Boost Resiliency

UNLOCKING THE MENTAL TRAP is a metaphor for how your choices and actions can free your mind from negative thoughts that prevent you from doing what you want. Moving away from isolation and loneliness may require learning how to slow down or speed up. You'll benefit from learning how to free your mind so you can engage in behaviours that increase your activity and energy.

Preparing your mind to unlock your mental trap helps shine a light on possibilities and generates hope. After years of counselling experience, I've discovered that when a person is open to change, they're positioned to learn how to take charge of their life.

Begin by becoming aware of what you can do, and then take accountability for your actions by committing to learn and practice new skills. By preparing to unlock your mental trap, you position yourself to shift fear, change any unwanted negative thoughts to positive ones, and experience more positive feelings.

Eliminate Bad Stress

A positive start is to practice daily to build up your resiliency, which can charge your mental battery so you have more energy to take on challenges. One key way is to recognize that stress can be helpful—but only to a point.

There are two types of stress: good stress and bad stress. Good stress motivates us. We need good stress to flourish and to perform to our full potential. Bad stress is any time we experience a difference between what we want and what we have. It can overwhelm us, and if it's chronic can make us ill.

Believing that no one could care for you or love you is an example of a painful thought that can be stressful. It's to your advantage to learn to effectively cope with such stressful thoughts.

You know what unwanted stress feels like, but did you know that stress accumulates over time and kills? Yes, stress kills! Stress can lead to heart attack and mental illness, like anxiety disorders. The longer you feel stress, the harder it is for your mind and body to cope and to stay healthy.

The Yerkes-Dodson law (aka the Inverted U-Model) teaches that performance will increase with mental arousal (stress) only up to a point. When you exceed this threshold, your performance decreases to the point that you can shut down.[1]

How you manage your emotions and thoughts under pressure determines how well you can regulate and stay in the optimal level of performance, called "the zone." In positive psychology, the zone refers to the flow state where you are fully engaged and involved, and is linked with positive feelings.[2] In this state, the task you're engaged in can seem easy and simple to do.

A person who's confident in their ability to make social connections and get along with others is more likely to be able

THE INVERTED U-MODEL

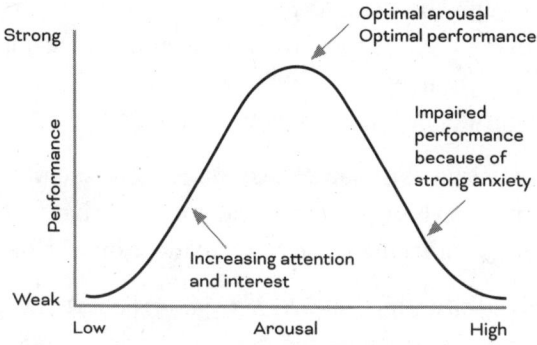

to engage in conversation than someone who's tense and worried about being accepted. Making new acquaintances can be stressful if you're not confident or are experiencing anxiety and fear. If you are preparing to unlock your mental trap, it's helpful to build up your resiliency skills so that you can better manage your emotions under pressure.

Let's look at what might happen when a person with weak resiliency skills faces a very stressful situation. James, who was married for 21 years, is experiencing a social connections disruption: his marriage has ended. Often, when a couple breaks up, one person appears to be more upset than the other; this person feels their heart has been broken. In James's case, he claims he never saw it coming. Is this possible? Perhaps. But why do people have affairs? Would James's wife, Sally, have engaged in another relationship if her current relationship with James was meeting her emotional needs? For a partner relationship to last, it takes two committed people who want to stay together. Sally's social connection with James was not strong enough to fill her need for love and belonging. She had a social connections gap around a personal relationship that likely included intimacy. Sally may have unintentionally found herself interacting with another man who helped her feel alive and excited. The opportunity resulted in emotions that led to an affair and her leaving her marriage for this new man.

Let's consider how James reacted to the breakup:

- **Trigger/situation:** James experiences a relationship breakup when his wife asks for a divorce. She has fallen in love with another man. She wants to move on with her life.

- **Perceived situation importance:** James believes he loves his wife and is in shock and disbelief when his wife tells him she's leaving. He never wanted this. This is a terrible life event for him.

- **Reaction to situation:** After the shock and experiencing lots of emotions, James blames himself—this is all his fault. He will not talk about it with family or friends. He begins to avoid people, as he feels embarrassed.

- **Resulting mental state:** James is depressed and unsure what his future will be like. He's isolating himself; he is drinking a bit more and paying less attention to his work. After two months, his stress level continues to be high.

> **Check-in**
>
> Put yourself in James's shoes and imagine how you would feel. Can you relate to how James reacted?

After two months, James is still in a crisis. He hasn't moved through the stages of grief; he's still in denial and anger.

James's anger is turning inward, causing him to pull away from his family and friends. The longer he isolates himself and uses this breakup as a reason to avoid and to fear trusting people, the more he puts his mental health at risk. As well, the hold his mental trap has on him strengthens, which can result in chronic negative thoughts and feelings that keep him more isolated and lonely.

Often in a situation like James's, there will be a period of grief. Many times, a person like James will move on after a period of typically two to six months. In some cases, a loss of a relationship that's perceived as traumatic can take much longer.

Resiliency Is a Trainable Skill

My first degree was in physical education and my classmates and I were taught the science of weight strength resistance, often called weightlifting. We were taught that the more a person can follow a structured weight resistance plan, the stronger they'll become over time. If they follow their plan, they also reduce their risk of injury. On the way to becoming stronger, it's common to have to push through discomfort to achieve a desired goal.

Like physical fitness, mental fitness requires intention. Focusing on building resiliency is a proven strategy to cope with day-to-day stressors. Life can be challenging, with good days and bad days. Nowhere are we promised that our lives will be filled with only good days.

I have heard the Dalai Lama speak, and he said that we should expect misery, and there's nothing good or bad about it. It's just the way it is. Miserable moments are akin to happy moments: they come and they go. The river of life can lead in many different directions. How you cope with your most stressful, challenging moments influences your outlook.

After one of my son's many breakups, sometime between the ages of 18 and 20, he asked me, "Dad, do you believe I'll be alone forever?"

"No," I said.

"Why?"

"I'm struggling to believe that out of the 7 billion people on this planet there's not another person who could like you and one you could like."

"I don't believe it."

"This lays out the problem."

"What do you mean?"

"It doesn't matter what I believe; it's what you believe. Sure, it makes sense that you're upset now. Grief is normal and healthy. But my response is about possibility, not timing."

I suspect you get the point that my son's emotions had overwhelmed him. What I found interesting was that by getting him in a conversation, asking questions, and providing some ideas, he moved from an emotionally charged state to a calmer state, because he was thinking consciously, not reacting unconsciously.

My questions created a cognitive bump that helped him take control of his emotions and consider possibility. This rejection taught him an important lesson that helped him develop his resiliency.

One way we develop resiliency is from life experiences. Failure, though painful, is a wonderful teacher. Failing provides an opportunity for new learning and personal growth. It's not fun, but when we're open and ready, we can learn from failure. It can teach us how to bounce back faster the next time we're faced with a similar challenge.

One of the biggest challenges with creating or maintaining a social connection is it takes two people who want the same thing. One person wanting to get to know someone isn't enough; the other person must want it, too. It's common for people to reject each other, and sometimes this creates emotional wounds that are difficult to move past.

When resiliency levels are low, pushing forward through a life challenge, such as a breakup, can take much longer than when resiliency levels are higher. A person with a low level of resiliency may think a breakup necessarily results in their feeling miserable for a long time. Researcher Paul Eastwick and his colleagues found that people often bounce back faster than they thought possible after a breakup.[3] This suggests that we often think things will be worse than they are. As well, our resiliency levels play a role in our ability to move through adversity. Your resiliency levels will be positively or negatively impacted by experiences with your environment.

Resiliency is a learned skill developed through life experiences, training, and practice. It can assist in dealing with life's adversity and setbacks. To be mastered, resiliency requires intention, focus, and practice. Buying a StairMaster alone will give you no physical exercise. To get the benefit, you must get on it and start moving. Resiliency is the same; just knowing what to do is not enough. You need to engage in mental fitness practices that have been proven to develop resiliency.

Charge Your Battery

Positive energy can come from a supportive manager, an attentive partner, or a caring friend. Energy drains can be negative peers, demanding work, a poor manager-employee relationship, or conflict with a family member. Not all energy drains are equal, but anything you perceive as stressful and unwanted is an energy drain. The more negative your experiences, the higher the drain on your resiliency.

Think of engaging in resiliency-building activities like charging a battery. What charges you is what you do with intention, such as exercise and mental fitness, and that you value and feel are a beneficial boost your resiliency.

> **Check-in**
>
> - What are your top three energy drains (i.e., stressors)?
> - What are the things you do to charge your battery?
> - What environmental factors do you have that help charge your battery (e.g., a pet)?

One of my biggest energy boosters is my dog, Dozer. He doesn't have to do a lot: whenever I'm around him, I feel better. He's so non-judgemental and caring; I feel better just being in his presence. I've learned how positive experiences—like being with Dozer—can have a positive impact on happiness. Savouring these moments allows me to create a bank of positive thoughts that I can draw upon to boost my thoughts and emotions. Research suggests that the more we practice savouring present and past moments, the more we positively impact our overall outlook on life.[4] Thinking about past social connections that you valued and enjoyed can help create positive thoughts. We can promote positive thoughts with intention.

Taking stock of all the good things you have can help your mental outlook. Researchers have found that practicing gratitude is good for your mental health and promotes happiness.[5] It's much easier to close social connections gaps when you have a positive outlook on what you have in your life.

Resiliency-Building Micro-Skills

The following micro-skills are meant to help you learn how to charge your battery by building resiliency. The more you charge your battery, the more energy you'll have to unlock your mental trap.

Develop Emotional Intelligence

Emotional intelligence (or EQ, emotional quotient) can help you develop your ability to manage your emotions under pressure. This psychological theory was developed by Peter Salovey and John Mayer, who defined emotional intelligence as "the ability to perceive emotions, to access and generate emotions so as to assist thought, to understand emotions and emotional knowledge, and to reflectively regulate emotions so as to promote emotional and intellectual growth."[6]

Becoming more mindful of your emotions—or becoming self-aware—can help you increase your EQ, which can lead to greater empathy for self and others; stronger ability to quiet the mind; and increased ease finding calm under pressure and staying composed. It becomes easier to gain perspective, so you aren't making decisions out of fear (such as the fear of rejection).

Consider for a moment how EQ can help you build social connections. People don't always get along, regardless of how much they care for or love each other. The conscious or unconscious expectation that things must always be calm and perfect in a relationship is not realistic. This expectation often leads to emotional pain when discord or disagreement arises.

"Things start out as hopes and end up as habits."

LILLIAN HELLMAN

Two people in conflict can have two separate points of view and both be right. Conflict is often not about right or wrong; it's about perspective, preferences, and priority. Individuals with lower EQ are less able to manage the fear and stress that come with conflict.

Imagine this scenario: you unlock your mental trap enough that you once again put yourself out there to make new social connections in the hopes of finding a new partner. After meeting a few people, you find someone with whom you'd like to go on a date. You go out on a few dates, and things seem to be going well. Then one night you have an argument. You don't see it coming; it happens on a phone call. Your fight or flight system fires off.

A person with high EQ will respond much differently to this situation than someone with low EQ. The high EQ person will dismiss any negative thinking quickly, put things in perspective, and treat the disagreement as not a big deal: "We'll cool down and chat tomorrow; all will be fine."

The low EQ individual will be more at risk of overreacting to this situation. They'll fear and believe they're going to be dumped and feel powerful emotions of depression, as well as feeling isolated and alone. This then can become a real problem. They may act out of fear and send texts that are all over the place emotionally, which become the reason the person now wants to dump them. Many times, it's not the event that breaks up couples. It's the perception of the event, followed by overreaching behaviour that creates or complicates an issue.

One of the fastest ways to build EQ is to become mindful and learn to observe your own emotions, thoughts, and behaviours. You can practice observing them daily in every interaction. Over time, with a mindful approach that focuses on what you're doing in the moment, you can develop your EQ.

Become familiar with the following EQ attributes.

- **Self-awareness** is the ability to be aware of your emotions and how they affect your thoughts and behaviours. An example is understanding the fight or flight system and learning how to better respond to perceived danger objectively. Your degree of self-awareness reflects how in tune you are with your strengths and weaknesses. This impacts your degree of self-confidence.

- **Relationship management** is your ability to develop and maintain healthy relationships by managing yourself. Relationship management skills are influenced by your ability to communicate with, influence, and motivate others; to work within a group; and to deal with conflict. If you have gaps in communication skills or conflict resolution, you can take a course. These are trainable skills that can help if you believe you would benefit from developing and practicing them.

- **Self-management** is the degree to which you can take charge of your impulsive feelings and behaviours and how effectively you manage yourself under pressure. Your ability to self-manage impacts your ability to take initiative without direction, follow through on commitments, and adapt to change.

- **Social awareness** is your ability to demonstrate empathy for others. Your degree of social awareness is determined by how well you can be in tune with and aware of others' emotions, needs, and concerns, as well as your ability to pick up on others' emotional cues, feel safe in social interactions, and manage power dynamics within social groups or at work.

Higher EQ can help reduce your risk of engaging in disruptive behaviours, such as saying things you don't mean, making kneejerk decisions that are regretted later, or damaging an important relationship because of your inability to control your emotions. The following tips can assist in developing your EQ:

- **Avoid emotional decisions:** The more connected you are to your emotions and how they can impact your daily decision making, the less likely you are to make decisions when you're emotionally overwhelmed. Adopt one simple rule: "I will not make a decision when I'm emotional because I don't want to make a poor one I'll regret later."

- **Practice empathy:** You likely want to feel valued at some level by yourself and others. Sometimes if you hyper-focus on your own needs, you can become somewhat self-absorbed. By noticing this and shifting your focus onto others' needs, you demonstrate empathy and compassion, which benefits others, feeds your sense of value, and supports developing higher EQ.

- **Read body language:** When you notice others' non-verbal cues, you're better able to adjust your message and social interactions. There's a well-known non-verbal communication rule called the 7/38/55 rule.[7] It suggests that 7 percent of the meaning of a communication comes from the words, 38 percent is in how the words are expressed, and 55 percent is expressed by body language. Understanding non-verbal communication is critical. Focusing on how the message is being communicated versus the message itself can provide the opportunity to build strong, trusted relationships.

- **Save 10 by taking 10:** It's amazing how 10 seconds of emotional discharge can take 10 hours or more to fix. When you're feeling emotionally charged, before you speak out of anger or fire off a response to a text or email, stop, pause, and regain your composure. Try taking 10 minutes to write out what you want to say. And then read it out loud to yourself, and consider how you'd take it if you were the one receiving that message.

There are many online courses and books available on EQ if you want to learn more. However, if you focus on the above tips and practice them, you may be surprised at how you can develop your EQ by focusing on it daily with mindful attention.

Learn Deep Breathing

One proven way to curb and reduce the negative impact of stress is deep breathing. Often referred to as diaphragmatic breathing, deep breathing brings more oxygen into the body.[8] The optimal time to use this micro-skill is when you're feeling anxious or stressed and want to feel like you're more in control. There are benefits to adding this practice to your daily routine as a tool to promote resiliency and mental health.

This skill requires little learning to gain its benefits. Read the following steps a few times, or record the instructions on your phone in a relaxing tone and pace, and then follow along as you play it back to yourself.

- Get comfortable in a quiet spot. It's fine to be sitting or lying down. If you choose to lie down, ensure your head is comfortable, and you're flat on your back with your legs pulled in and your knees bent up.

- Rest one open, flat hand above your belt line, facing palm down, and the other palm down on your upper chest. Your hands are guides to show you which parts of your body are moving up and down as you breathe. When doing deep breathing, the top hand is not to move.

- This deep breathing exercise begins with a gentle exhale. There's no need to empty your lungs. This action is meant only to prepare for the deep breathing exercise. As you lightly exhale, let your body rest by allowing your neck and shoulders to relax.

- After you have exhaled, close your mouth, and pause for a second. Think about being relaxed.

- When you're ready to begin, slowly breathe in through your nose and fill your lungs. Focus on bringing the air deep into your lungs so that your belly and bottom hand rise. The upper hand will not move, only the bottom hand as you breathe in deeply. Bring in as much air as you can comfortably.

- Hold this air in for a minimum of five seconds. The length of time will be determined by your level of comfort.

- Slowly and gently release the air through your mouth. Continue to do so until you've released all the air that you can. As you breathe out, imagine all your stress is riding a wave away from you, and feel the tension leave your body.

- Once all the air is out, pause, and close your mouth. Prepare to repeat the deep breathing cycle.

- Repeat this cycle, one breath at a time. Do this five to seven times in each practice session.

Practice Cognitive Hygiene

The average person has 50,000 to 70,000 thoughts per day; that's around 35 to 48 per minute.[9] With this much mental activity, it's normal to have moments when you feel overwhelmed or distracted. More problematic are negative thoughts about yourself. When these thoughts are left unchecked and become repetitive and ingrained, they can negatively impact your perceptions, decisions, and actions, both at work and home.

Be clear of the value and reason that it's in your best interest to practice cognitive hygiene every day. Did you have any negative thoughts about yourself today, such as, "I'm weak; I'm a failure; I'm no good; no one likes me"? Sadly, these kinds of automatic thoughts are quite normal. It's what you do with them that's important. Negative thoughts can grow, and when left unchecked, they can erode your mental health and strengthen your mental trap.

Like brushing your teeth routinely to deal with bacteria before it builds up, it's much easier to clean out a day's worth of negative thoughts than to ignore them and deal with the consequences six months down the road. Accountability is owning what you can directly control: your thinking. Begin by flagging negative thoughts and acknowledging that they're not helpful. Practice making this statement to yourself: "This thought isn't helpful to my health and happiness, so it can go." Many unwanted thoughts are automatic, and with practice they can be removed as quickly as they form. Owning your thoughts positions you to move from being the observer to the driver of what you think. The more you practice cognitive hygiene, the better you'll be at dismissing unwanted thoughts.

The following approach may help you get on track to turn off stubborn, unwanted thoughts:

- Write out the thought on a piece of paper.
- Consider why you're having this thought now. Did someone say it to you? Is it based on personal or work experience? Or are you not sure?
- In a safe and quiet spot, read the thought out loud.
- Write out the emotions that are associated with this thought.
- On a scale of 1 (low) to 10 (high), how true do you believe this thought is?
- Try to understand how the thought is impacting you.
- Is there anything stopping you from turning off this thought and accepting that it's not in your best interest?
- For stubborn thoughts that you believe you can't simply turn off, repeat the above process for three days. Write in a daily journal to trap the thoughts.
- If after three days you can't remove the unwanted thought and it's causing you stress, anxiety, or depression, you may benefit from professional support. It's normal to feel apprehensive or to feel the stigma related to these thoughts. One in five Canadians is at mental health risk. Of the individuals at risk, only one out of three seeks professional help.[10] Bring the work you've done to a professional counsellor to help them understand your experience and challenge.

Try Cognitive Reframing

Cognitive reframing is a micro-skill that can be learned quite easily, but it requires a desire to take accountability for your negative thinking. It positions you to change your negative thoughts by considering positive alternatives. For example, a negative thought about work, such as "The project ending suddenly without notice or any input on what we accomplished is not what I wanted," can be positively reframed: "But I did get to spend four months on a project I enjoyed, and I've had a chance to demonstrate my skills." Cognitive reframing can teach you how to change your perspective and that in turn can impact your thinking, emotions, and actions. Here are some tips for cognitive reframing:

- **Believe:** Benefitting from this micro-skill starts with the belief that you can't control all the events in your world, but you can control how you react to them.

- **Identify opportunities for cognitive reframing:** When you become aware of internal dialogue that's creating a negative view of yourself, your world, or your future, recognize it as an opportunity to try changing the script.

- **Accept that negative thoughts can go as quickly as they come:** One way to reduce the influence of negative thinking is to change your focus quickly. As fast as a negative thought appears, it can be replaced by changing the context: "What would you tell your best friend if they were in the same situation as you're in now?" You too can benefit from the positive alternatives you would create for others. You need only listen.

- **Focus energy on the positive alternative story:** Look for ways to change your story into a positive one, which can improve how you're thinking and feeling.

Rewire Your Brain to Find Positivity

Rick Hanson, a neuropsychologist and bestselling author, reported that we're evolutionarily wired to notice bad over good.[11] This made sense 200,000 years ago when our ancestors were trying to avoid threats and survive. Neuroplasticity refers to the brain's ability to reorganize itself and change its hardwiring structures over our lifetime.[12] This can be both positive and negative for our mental health. If you're not aware that your brain has a natural bias to notice negativity first, and you don't know that you can train it to see more positively, you risk becoming more prone to focusing on negativity. This can impact your thinking, emotions, and general mental health. As negativity becomes more intense, it can result in increased risk of mental illness, such as depression.

Understanding this basic brain research helps to promote positive action to offset thinking patterns that promote negative plasticity.[13] With proper treatment and support, you can learn to stop the negativity and repair your brain so it can become more positively wired. This is the micro-skill of thinking of the positives first. When you walk into a situation, approach it with the intention of looking for the positive. By being aware that your brain is naturally biased, and reminding yourself of that and refocusing, you can train it to find the positive first. If you've been overly prone to see the negative first and have a difficult time seeing the positive, you can change this with intention and practice. As with the lessons learned in meditation, this micro-skill benefits from being patient while learning it and not judging yourself; just notice your thoughts and then gently refocus your attention on the positive.

For this micro-skill to work, it's necessary to understand and accept that only you can directly increase your positive brain plasticity. If you are struggling to do it alone, professionals can help you learn how. Positive change begins with awareness and requires self-motivation. Committing to finding more of the positives in your life can benefit your mental health over time. Your brain's wiring is impacted by your habitual thinking. The more you create positive plasticity, the more likely you'll wire more happiness into your brain. Here are some tips to practice:

- **Search for the positives:** Before you walk into your home, commit that you'll notice three positives before allowing your brain to focus on a negative—for instance, first notice a birthday card from a friend, a bouquet of flowers, and freshly washed floors, rather than focusing on the garbage you need to take out. You can apply this practice to work, team sports, and relationships. If your brain goes to a negative, don't judge it; release it and move on to find the positive.

- **Give the positive more airtime and importance:** It's common when people get together for them to talk about what's not working and focus on negatives. Commit to giving the positives more airtime when you interact with others. By focusing on the positive and talking about it, you create conditions and expectations for your brain to notice more positives, so you have more to share. This activity can also influence others to think positively, which will help them as well.

- **Refocus on the solution:** Life isn't perfect, so there will be times when you face a challenge that you want to be over and done with. The key is to move away from negative thinking because it inhibits you from finding a solution. By acknowledging the challenge and changing your focus to finding a solution—a positive—you move your attention away from your brain's fear centre to activate its other parts that drive decision making and planning. This helps to increase your resiliency and move through life's challenges and setbacks.

Practice Three-Minute Meditation

Your mind may be filled to the brim with to-do lists for tasks at work and home, and perhaps you're inundated with information at every turn—from the TV or your smartphone or email—and you're facing constant interruptions. Your mind can get overloaded and you risk losing the ability to focus and to manage your emotions with this mental chaos.

Fortunately, there's a way to find a few moments of quiet for your mind that can have a huge impact on your resiliency. Meditation is an activity that continues to gain attention as an effective strategy for promoting resiliency. Here are tips for meditating:

- **Develop a practice:** One easy practice is called focused-attention meditation, where all you need is a quiet, safe spot where you can focus on meditation for three minutes. The practice requires you to place your attention on a single object, breath, sound, or visualization. Choose a safe spot and prepare yourself to meditate. Open the stopwatch on your smartphone. Pick your focus point (e.g., a spot on the floor, the sensation of your breath). Start your stopwatch. Move your attention to your focus point and begin meditating. When your mind wanders, which it will, don't judge. Be patient and bring attention back to your focus. When you think you've done at least three minutes, stop. Look at your timer to see how you've done. The more you practice, three minutes will fly by and you may find you go longer, which is fine.

- **Set a daily expectation:** For the next 90 days, set a goal to meditate for three minutes a day, and commit to when you'll do it (e.g., when you wake up or just before going to sleep).

Visualize Mindfully

Through the power of focus and attention, you can influence and reshape your brain's architecture.[14] Neuroplasticity research indicates that it takes the same level of effort to become a worrier as it does to become calm. Mindful visualization is a structured model designed to facilitate mindfulness that can influence how you view and interact with the world. Creating experiences that promote calm and happiness can shape the brain, so it improves its ability to be calm and happy, benefitting your experiences both at work and at home. Here's how to do it:

- **Measure your current state:** On a scale of 1 (not calm at all) to 5 (very calm), how calm are you? Write this number in your daily calendar so you can track it.

- **Find now:** Look around and notice five things that you can hear or see (e.g., the colour of your shoes, a clock, the sound of a fan). This transition step gets your mind from where it was to now.

- **Take five:** Practice being in the moment without judgement for five minutes. Use a timer or go by feel. It's fine to go a bit longer but not less. To prepare for this step, take a few gentle breaths in and out to relax and then set your eyes on a spot. Allow your mind to be empty and just focus on your breathing or the spot you're looking at. If your mind wanders off task, that's fine; just bring it back to now and focus on the spot. This mindful step helps train your brain to slow down. It gets easier with practice.

- **Visualize benefits:** Some people, when they visualize, can run a mental video; others hear an audio story. It doesn't matter. As above, no judgement: when your mind wanders, catch yourself and come back to your visualization. Visualize yourself being calm in situations you find challenging or worry about. Picture yourself in different situations where you can stay calm. We've all seen others stay calm under pressure. Use this as a reference point to fill in the blanks for your visualization. Focus only on success and positives—no negatives. If a negative jumps into your mind, release it. Think about what you did in the visualization. How did others react? The outcome of visualization is experiencing the benefits of being calm and thinking about how a calm person behaves, thinks, and feels.

- **Anchor success:** Using the same scale from the first step, remeasure how calm you are. Track your progress over the next six weeks. Once you master this exercise, you can replace calm with any quality you choose to add to your life, such as happiness.

Journal to Process Day-to-Day Stress

Journaling at the end of your day to process the day's events is an effective micro-skill that can help manage stress and emotions. Journaling can vary from writing your thoughts in a notebook to filling in a daily log that tracks your resiliency, physical activities, and emotions. Emotional tracking helps you pay attention to your mood trends. Journaling creates a catalogue and record of your days that you can use to see how you're doing and the progress you've made over time.

One study found that people tend to be more upset about losing $50 than they are happy about gaining $50.[15] Positive psychology leaders like Shawn Achor, who did a TEDxBloomington talk viewed by more than 22 million people, promote the need for people to focus less on what's negative in life and more on what's positive. Achor promotes the value of investing energy in our social network and to take stock daily of three things we're grateful for to foster a positive attitude. If we do this, we can improve our mental map, learn to view the world more positively, and become happier. Journaling is an effective approach for promoting well-being and for processing emotions and increasing self-awareness.[16]

You have lots of data coming at you every day in many different forms, from the internet, social media, and emails. Keeping up with that amount of information can feel overwhelming. Prospect theory teaches that your desire to avoid negative experiences is stronger than your desire to take action to obtain positive experiences. You own your mental health, but it can be difficult, especially without a frame of reference to understand what you can do to take charge and reduce the risk of putting more focus on negative over positive events.

One study found that people who journaled on average 20 minutes a day before surgery were able to recover faster than those who did not.[17] The research found that the act of writing about stressful events can help a person see stress as a challenge, not a hindrance. Journaling doesn't need to be complicated. It's simply taking the words out of your head and recording them so you take a moment to process what you're thinking. This self-awareness can help you feel more in control and balanced. Many of my clients journal. In fact, I wrote a couple of journaling guides—*Journal 45* and *Journal 51*. Some clients told me that within a few weeks they noticed a positive benefit from journaling five to 10 minutes a day and recording their dominant emotions for the day.

You'll have good days and challenging ones; that's just the reality of being a human. You likely haven't been taught or raised to understand that a bad day is nothing more than a point in time, and like good days, it too shall pass.

It's helpful to be able to dismiss bad moments quickly to ensure you don't adopt them as being a dominant representation of your life. Keeping a daily journal with a daily log can help track emotions and allow you to keep perspective.

- **Start a daily journal:** You can use pen and paper, you may elect to write out your daily thoughts electronically, or you may decide to purchase one of the many online journaling tools available. Processing each day's events in a journal can help you close out your day on a positive note so that you start the next day with a clean slate. I've been a fan of daily journaling for a long time, as it can be a wonderful way to keep an objective perspective.

- **Keep a daily emotional log:** I recommend as a part of your daily journaling that you consider completing a daily emotional log. At the end of each day, reflect on the emotions you experienced and file them in your emotional log. It's helpful to keep the perspective that one or two days is not a trend. However, constantly feeling sad for two weeks is. A daily log of your emotions works like a dashboard on a car when a warning light tells you it's time to pull over and make an adjustment. In the case of emotions, the adjustment is to challenge your thinking.

- **Note chargers and disruptions:** Each day, take a minute to note which charging and disrupting emotions you experienced at home and work. Examples of life-charging emotions are loving, happy, grateful, valued, relaxed, peaceful, confident, satisfied, joy. Examples of life-disrupting emotions include anxious, angry, depressed, hopeless, empty, rejected, guilty, sad, and fear.

- **Keep a daily well-being log:** Some daily micro-habits provide energy that charge your mental battery, just as positive social connections do. Like a daily emotional record, this is a simple log to keep. I've seen first-hand how intention and daily focus in these areas can help charge one's battery and build mental fitness and resiliency levels. Consider how positive you believe each area was for you, how much you feel it charged your battery that day. The more you focus on each area and make it a priority, the more likely it will be a positive for you. The higher the score from 1 (low) to 10 (high), the more this area has been positive for the day.

- **Sleep:** had a good night's sleep
- **Nutrition:** paid attention to diet
- **Exercise:** moved with intention to be physically active
- **Relax:** took time to relax
- **Passion:** engaged my passion (e.g., hobby, sport, volunteering)
- **Social connections:** engaged with intention to strengthen and maintain connections
- **Family (if applicable):** had a positive day with family
- **Partner (if applicable):** had a loving day

Set Personal Goals

One proven method for developing resiliency to support your mental fitness is personal goal setting. Setting a goal without clarity on how you'll achieve it often results in failure. Wanting something and not planning how to achieve it is a common mistake. Wanting to be happy makes sense, but what you're going to do differently to become happy must be thought through.

There are many different goal-setting methods out there, such as SMART goals. This acronym stands for specific, measurable, achievable, relevant, and time-bound. The purpose of a SMART goal is to obtain clarity on what you'll do, how, and when. When a goal is clear and simple, it's easier to achieve and measure. When setting a SMART goal, first answer the question of *why* you want the desired outcome. It's helpful to not just say you want to meet more people and build more social connections: you need to be clear *why* that matters to you. When you have a clear, meaningful *why* and see the benefit of the outcome, this increases your motivation and solidifies your intention to achieve the goal.

There's a line of research that suggests setting a goal is as important as considering what may prevent the goal from becoming a reality. This is a method called mental contrast, where you begin by visualizing what you want, followed by the obstacles. An evidence-based goal-setting model called WOOP (which stands for wish, outcome, obstacle, plan), developed in the field of positive psychology, appears to be an effective way to set goals.[18] The neat thing about WOOP is you can use it for small daily goals or for larger longer-term goals. I like it, as it's straightforward and can be used on demand. Here is a six-step process that uses the WOOP model. I've found it useful for helping people achieve their goals.

1. **Find five minutes of quiet:** Before beginning, be mindful, slow down, clear your mind, and relax. The goal of this step is to find some calm.

2. **Wish:** What do you want to achieve? Think about something in your life that you want to achieve. For example, make a better social connection in the workplace.

3. **Outcome:** What is the most desirable outcome? If you achieve this goal, visualize how it will help you and what

the benefit will be for you. Think about what you expect this outcome will do for your overall sense of well-being and happiness.

4. **Obstacle:** What are some obstacles to achieving this goal? Think about the things that could make this goal hard to achieve, and then what options you have to work around them. If obstacles arise, what would you do? Picture yourself working through these obstacles to your goal.

5. **Plan:** Plan as to how and when you'll begin to achieve your goal. Include in the plan some "If X happens, I'll do Y" strategies. Think about what you can do to get from point A to point B. Consider the different what-if situations, so that in the event you face some challenges, you are prepared.

6. **Write out your plan and how you'll measure success:** Once you plan your goal, write it down. Putting a goal on paper helps to reinforce it and increases your accountability. You can add a daily measurement of progress toward your goal in your journal. Increase your accountability by telling any trusted friends or family members what you're trying to achieve. Often when we make things public, it increases our social accountability to others and ourselves.

The sooner you become comfortable with goal setting, the better. One major goal to set if your mental trap is holding you in a negative mindset is learning how to unlock it. No matter what degree of struggle you might have unlocking your mental trap, in order to be successful you'll need to be intentional and set clear goals along your journey—and then take action.

Check-in

- Start practicing one micro-skill today.

- Consider adopting journaling as one of your daily behaviours to promote resiliency, as it is a skill we'll leverage later in building social connections. Start practicing now as you work your way through the process laid out in this book.

- Following a structured plan can help build the confidence and competency needed to achieve a desired goal—in this case, to move away from isolation and loneliness.

- Start setting WOOP goals with intention. An example may be to charge your mental battery to give you more energy and resources to push through any challenges you face on your way to closing social connections gaps.

Tips to Promote Resiliency

You'll notice that intention is at the core of all the micro-skills. Without intention and practice, you'll have little opportunity to benefit from them. The following 40 tips are meant to demonstrate that if you just notice and do a bit more here and there, you can increase your resiliency. The goal is to charge your battery so you're prepared and in the best mental state possible to unlock your mental trap.

"Social acceptance, 'being liked,' has so much power because it holds the feelings of loneliness at bay."

ROLLO MAY

- **Improve your self-acceptance:** Decide to focus on learning to accept yourself. When you accept yourself, you're more likely to believe others will accept you.

- **Start intrinsic motivation:** You must want to leave isolation and loneliness behind, and be open to the fact that to do so will require you to learn how to make healthy choices that promote building social connections.

- **Recognize that social connections are important:** Decide to improve your social connections because they're important. Learn how to meet and trust people who have skills, resources, and ideas different from yours. Consider taking a course on building personal networks to develop social skills and meet people.

- **Define your life purpose:** Write out exactly what you want your life purpose to be, as well as how you want to be remembered when you die.

- **Be compassionate:** Extend compassion to yourself and others, with the goal of easing suffering. Caring for others can provide meaningful experiences and the motivation to be with other people.

- **Adopt integrity thinking:** Write out your core values and pay attention to them daily. Decide that you'll live your life and make decisions that are aligned with your life purpose and core values.

- **Focus on your mental fitness:** Use micro-skills such as mindfulness, deep breathing, and meditation that are excellent for calming your mind and creating mental space. Build a mental fitness plan that supports your quest to build new social connections and find more authentic connections. Mental fitness will provide you with the resiliency required to be successful.

- **Find authentic connections in your life:** Think of a relationship—present or in the past—that is genuine, safe, caring, honest, and trusting, and where you can be vulnerable and feel comfortable being yourself in a way that brings you and another person joy.

- **Perform acts of kindness:** Engage in random acts of kindness that help others. Kindness creates a "helper's high" that can promote a desire in you to interact more with others. It will also create positive energy, which people want to be around.

- **Evaluate your current relationships:** Examine your relationships to see if you're unclear on how to define roles, rules, and expectations and if they're breaching your values. Negative, judgemental people can bring you down. To move forward and find peace and happiness, you may need to end some toxic relationships.

- **Practice unplugging:** Track your screen time and time spent on social media. Set goals to scale back so you have time for authentic relationships, which take time and commitment.

- **Practice being present with others:** When interacting with others, focus on what the other person is saying by paying attention, listening, and asking questions. People are attracted to those who are caring and supportive. They're likely to reciprocate attention.

- **Show up:** Don't take relationships for granted. Accept that to have authentic relationships, you have to be available, invest energy in learning about the other person, and give them time to learn about you.

- **Improve your social connections:** Consider making an effort to invest energy and time in getting to know others in person, and continue to develop those friendships.

- **Take care of your physical fitness:** What's good for the body is good for the mind. It's helpful to be active, eat well, stay hydrated, and make well-balanced lifestyle decisions (e.g., if you drink alcohol, do so moderately).

- **Set work boundaries:** Define when work will stop and start so that you can engage in relationships outside work with predictability.

- **Monitor personal health and happiness regularly:** Pay attention to your daily stress levels to monitor patterns of feeling overloaded. Use an app that tracks daily emotions and has a journaling feature, so you foster positive habits and avoid developing negative ones.

- **Accept that you don't have to do this alone:** We all want to have strong social connections. Know that you're not alone, and your journey doesn't need to be travelled alone. If you're struggling to make progress, consider working with a mental health professional who will support you. There's nothing wrong with getting professional help to explore your life options and challenges.

- **Energy will come in time:** It's normal to feel discouraged when trying to change behaviours. Retraining your brain takes energy, practice, and patience. As the adage goes, inch by inch, life can be a cinch. It begins with one step, one day at a time.

- **Be open to group initiatives:** Participate in employer or community events designed to bring people together.

- **Plan fun activities:** Engaging in fun activities that are healthy and safe can have a positive impact on your emotional state. Make a plan to add more humour and joy to your life.

- **Pick happiness over pleasure:** Be clear that happiness is forever. All you need to do to experience it is focus on a time when you were happy to get the benefit. Pleasure can be addictive and short-term. Pleasure can create the illusion of fulfillment, but it's only temporary. Focus on things that create happiness.

- **Recognize the power of a pet:** Pets whom we love know only one thing—how to love us back. They're consistent and caring and can create powerful, healthy connections.

- **Share your talents with others:** Most of us have gifts and talents; the challenge is how to share them with others. There can be a great deal of joy in helping others.

- **Manage your brain's natural drugstore:** Dopamine is a feel-good neurotransmitter that your brain releases when you engage in something you enjoy. It can be as small as going for a daily walk.

- **Know there's no such thing as perfection:** Remove the burden or expectation that you should be perfect. Consider that life will have imperfections.

- **Accept that moving from loneliness requires change:** Be ready to face any resistance (e.g., internal voices and excuses); nothing will change unless you do.

- **Sleep:** Make sleep important; consistently getting a good night's sleep improves your mental state and motivation.

- **Be clear that loneliness is a feeling, not a fact:** Loneliness is often triggered by a feeling, not by isolation. The brain hyper-focuses on the negative emotion, but loneliness is not a permanent state.

- **Resist faulty programming:** Negative thinking (e.g., "I'm a social outcast") can trigger decisions to withdraw into yourself, which makes your feeling of loneliness more intense.

- **Focus outward:** Shift your attention from yourself to the outside world, which can bring relief and move you away from feelings of isolation and loneliness.

- **Find others like you:** Consider how you could meet people who are interested in things you enjoy. There are clubs for pretty much every hobby and interest. Finding people who share your passions can create new social connections.

- **Be curious:** Challenging yourself to engage in social connections feeds your curiosity and creativity to problem-solve and can help you to create a situation where you'll find success.

- **Adopt persistence:** It may take five or more social connections experiments to find one that feels right. Accept that part of the process of finding strong social connections is walking away from weak ones.

- **Explore online peer groups:** Online peer support resources like Togetherall can help you meet people, share your concerns, or ask questions in a safe, confidential place.

- **Explore happiness:** Define what happiness means for you and how you will know you're happy. Create a happiness list of the top 10 things you do that make you happy. Even if you haven't done something in a while, like skating or swimming, if they made you happy in the past and you can physically do them today, they likely will make you happy again.

- **Be aware of the power of micro-social touches:** There's a line of research that suggests that we get a boost of happiness by just saying hello to strangers.[19] This suggests that human beings feel better by being more social. Try saying hello to strangers that you don't get a negative feeling from.

- **Share experiences with others:** One way to build and strengthen social connections is to share experiences.[20] People tend to enjoy hearing stories about experiences, which helps them expand their own experience and to relate to you. This is where common interest and common ground can come from.

- **Be careful about assuming what others think:** One thing most humans do well, ironically, is mispredicting what others think, feel, and want.[21] Be careful making assumptions that can feed self-doubt. You don't know anything for certain until a person tells you what they're thinking.

- **Remember that undetected loneliness is a major health concern:** Becoming lonely and trapped in loneliness, especially when you're older or more vulnerable, can lead to premature death.[22] For greater self-awareness, measure your loneliness with a validated loneliness scale (e.g., Howatt HR's Loneliness Quick Survey[23] or the UCLA Loneliness Scale[24]). These tools can help you gain perspective as to why you feel the way you do. Loneliness can be treated through closing social connections gaps.

> **Check-in**
>
> - Pick three of the above tips that you most relate to and like.
>
> - Consider focusing on them and journal daily how they're helping you.
>
> - The more we practice these tips with intention, the more we can shape how we view the world. It begins with awareness, motivation, and conviction to practice. Like with any skill, the more you practice, the faster you'll master it and reap its benefits.

Building social connections can appear impossible when you're overwhelmed by negative thoughts that fill you with self-doubt. Learning to uncover the possibility of self-acceptance is one step in the journey to building new social connections. Healthy social connections are a source of energy that can charge your battery. It's also important to accept that no one can make you happy if you're not happy within.

My experience in teaching resiliency is that if you're focused and practice building your resiliency with intention (e.g., adopting two micro-skills such as journaling, deep breathing, mindfulness, three-minute meditation practice daily), you'll improve your mental fitness. Even after you learn to unlock your mental trap, it's a good idea to keep practicing, to keep developing your mental fitness. Remember the four pillars for mental health: physical health, mental fitness, social connections, and environmental factors. In the next chapter, we'll explore how your current mental trap may be preventing you from closing social connections gaps, and you'll discover frameworks to support you.

7

Framing to Unlock Your Mental Trap

AT THE CORE of unlocking the mental trap is self-control. Self-control facilitates goals such as losing weight and intentionally building more social connections. On the journey to achieving goals, it's common to experience setbacks and failures that can deplete your confidence and inner strength. When hit by a challenging moment, people tend to slip back to old, comfortable patterns. That's why building a framework first is important.

Two systems in the brain influence your degree of self-control and drive toward a desired goal. The behavioural activation system (BAS) supports you in moving toward a goal and the behavioural inhibition system (BIS) cautions you against moving toward a goal.[1] Think of these as the gas and brake pedals in a car. Building resiliency and motivation is important to keep your BAS activated and engaged.

"We often think ourselves into problems. To get out of them requires us to keep thinking": this is a go-to line I've used many times in my counselling career. It's meant to set the stage and to normalize that we often—without realizing it—think in a way that's not in our best interest. Many of my clients are surprised to discover that their negative thoughts are coming from within, and no one on the outside is making them have those thoughts; it's how they're processing their experience. In these conversations, the client gets to witness how their emotional and psychological pain comes from their mind, and it's their negative thinking that's contributing to this misery.

If your mental trap is stopping, inhibiting, or distracting you, the first goal is to increase self-awareness, followed by a desire and readiness to take charge of thinking. Unlocking mental traps is about learning how to stop unwanted, negative thoughts and then replace them with more positive and empowering ones. Knowledge is power, and once you have insights that can positively change your thinking, you'll be one step closer to unlocking your mental trap.

Values Framework

Motivation to change begins with personal core values. It's common for a person to be unaware of their core values. Why? They're operating on autopilot, with their primary focuses on their job, paying bills, and taking care of family responsibilities. Your core values impact what you prioritize and what motivates you. To learn how to close social connections gaps, you'll benefit from making mental health a core value. To make any change to your mental health requires intention, and you must rank mental health as important as family or work.

> **Check-in**
>
> - List your top three personal core values.
> - Did you put your mental health on this list?

Happiness Framework

It was once thought that your happiness set-point was fixed. This is the level of happiness you return to after a wonderful experience when you're elated, or after moving through a negative experience. Neuroplastic research has found that when you intentionally practice to change your thoughts and feelings, you can rewire your brain and teach it to find more internal happiness and calm. What's amazing is how fast you can get results.[2] As little as 12 weeks of practice and focus on your thoughts and feelings can have a positive impact on how you view the world and yourself.

Self-Awareness Framework

The following elements will help increase your self-awareness, as you prepare to unlock your mental trap.

My Experience with Loneliness

Loneliness is often a by-product of perceived isolation. Feeling lonely is a normal emotion, and typically a sign that you're experiencing a social connections gap. The uncomfortable feeling of being lonely can inspire you to reach out, such as by texting, emailing, or calling someone. It's like being thirsty is a signal from your body that you're missing something. In the case of thirst, it's fluid, which you can remedy by drinking. However, when you're unable to close your social connections gap because of your mental trap, feelings of loneliness continue. The longer there's a gap, the greater the risk of experiencing loneliness. The antidote for loneliness is meaningful, authentic social connections.

- On a scale of 1 (low) to 10 (high), how concerned are you on a typical day about feeling isolated?
- On a scale of 1 (low) to 10 (high), how concerned are you on a typical day about feeling lonely?

My Primary Daily Emotions

Moving from loneliness to closing social connections gaps is not like flipping a switch. It's a process, which means there can be moments when things seem grey and bleak that test you. In these moments, it's helpful to leverage your resiliency micro-skills (e.g., deep breathing) that calm your mind. Being aware of the link between your thoughts, emotions, and mood provides insight into what's happening.

- Reflect over the past 90 days what a typical day looks like for you in terms of the percentage of the day that has positive versus negative emotions. Don't worry about being right; take a guess. For example, 60 percent positive and 40 percent negative.
- What you believe to be your most dominant emotion will dominate your mood. In one sentence, how would you describe your mood over the past few months?

My Cognitive Schemas

As discussed earlier, negative cognitive schemas filter how you interpret the world.

- What's one negative cognitive schema that has influenced how you experience social connections? Complete the following sentence: "I am…"

- When you say this to yourself, what emotions are attached? Notice the link between your thoughts and emotions.

My Fear

When we are overwhelmed by fear, we can perceive a loss of control and perspective. Understanding your fight or flight response system allows you to be more objective so that you can respond to non-lethal danger with a proportional response.

- Think of a situation where your fight or flight response system fired off when you knew there was no real danger. How often does this happen?

- What are the consequences when this happens?

My Ability to Manage Emotions Under Pressure

Through mindful practice, you can learn how to not overreact to negative emotions. Naming the emotion and acknowledging it can help you gain perspective in times of stress. Emotions are just feelings that are connected to some level of thinking that may or may not be true.

- On a scale of 1 (low) to 10 (high), how confident are you on a typical day that you can manage your emotions under pressure?

- Can you remember a situation in which you overreacted, and your reaction made the situation more stressful than it needed to be?

The primary objective of the above activity is to bring to your level of awareness how much your mental trap may be impacting your day-to-day choices. Insight into how you deal with stress can help you become aware of how strong your mental trap is.

The stronger its hold, the more you will be concerned or unsure that you will be able to unlock your mental trap. Be clear that you have already started with self-awareness, which is a valuable first step. Your level of commitment, motivation, and desire to learn will define your effort to unlock your mental trap. As you learn to control your mental trap, not only will you be able to close social connections gaps, but you'll also be better able to make decisions about your career, finances, and physical health.

Leveraging Cognitive-Behavioural Approach (CBA) Concepts

People use different kinds of counselling techniques to unlock their mental traps. One that has lots of scientific support for helping change negative thinking and emotions is the cognitive-behavioural approach (CBA). This form of psychology was developed to help people better understand and learn how to unlock their mental traps, as well as believe they can learn how to be happier.

Practicing CBA can help you gain perspective on how your automatic thoughts and emotions can fool you into believing things that often aren't true. For example, an automatic thought, such as "I'm not loveable," is nothing more than a thought. There's no evidence; it's just an unconscious, randomly generated thought. However, what matters is the power we give the thought. The power defines how the thought will shape feelings and behaviours. If the thought is allowed to keep playing over and over like an audio loop, over time it can erode self-confidence.

Your brain is a wonderful machine, but when you don't have the instructions on how it works, in challenging times it can take you down the wrong path. CBA provides insight into how to influence thoughts, emotions, and behaviours.

To benefit from CBA, much like having good physical health, requires intention and action to obtain a desired outcome. How long it will take for the following three-step CBA model to help you unlock your mental trap can vary. But in some cases, the activities in this section may be enough to loosen or even unlock your mental trap. The goal is to help you discover new perspectives to better manage negative thinking and emotions.

Learning how to unlock your mental trap begins with acknowledging that negative thinking and emotions are holding you back from engaging in the kinds of social connections you want. There are no shortcuts or magic wands. Making personal change requires effort, time, patience, and sometimes dealing with some personal discomfort—no different than if you hurt your leg in a car accident and had to go to physiotherapy to get it back to its full potential. These exercises can be challenging, but the reward is getting your leg back in operation.

Step 1: Frame Your Mental Trap

Keep in mind that closing social connections gaps is a process. It can take time, and sometimes a desire for things to happen fast can result in pushing too hard and pushing others away.

One realistic expectation is to learn how to become comfortable with yourself. Know who you are, what makes you tick, and what makes you happy. Be clear about your strengths and gaps. It's often helpful building relationships with people who are aligned with your core values but may have different strengths and skills.

Take time to ponder each set of questions. Your answers will help you learn to what degree your mental trap may be impacting your feelings, thoughts, expectations, and behaviours.

Feelings: What kinds of feelings are you experiencing, concerning social connections gaps, isolation, and loneliness? List in your own words the top three feelings that come up when you think about your experience with social connections gaps, isolation, and loneliness.

Thoughts: Your mental trap represents your current views about the quality of social connections at home, at work, and in your community. Take some time to consider the following questions: How hopeful are you that you'll be able to close your social connections gaps? Do you believe you can trust another person? Do you see a benefit in having an authentic partnership connection? Is it possible any of your current negative thinking around social connections could be wrong?

Expectations: Your thoughts can be influenced by your expectations—what you think you should have in your life. As you challenge your thoughts, it's helpful to also be mindful that your expectations influence what you'll define as being good or bad. It's important to set realistic expectations as well as to be open to change your expectations as you discover and learn about yourself and the people you meet. Flexibility without compromising core values is a valuable part of learning how to build relationships. What does success look like for you in the short term regarding closing social connections gaps?

Behaviours: Feelings and thoughts can influence behavioural choices. What coping behaviours that you engage in are you most concerned about? What behaviours would you like to be doing?

Step 2: Explore the Impact of Worrying

Worry can be a helpful emotion when it reminds you of what you need and influences you to get something done to address that concern. For example, your gas tank is low on fuel. Worry reminds you to get the tank filled so you don't run out, and it keeps poking you until you fill the tank. This is helpful. But if your tank is full and you keep worrying, that's not helpful.

It helps to know that worry serves some purpose: it can identify a concern or problem. It's normal to worry and impossible to eliminate all worry. Worry becomes a concern when it's miswired and goes on for too long. If you don't see a solution to a problem and allow worry to continue, it can become overwhelming and turn into a three-part negative loop.

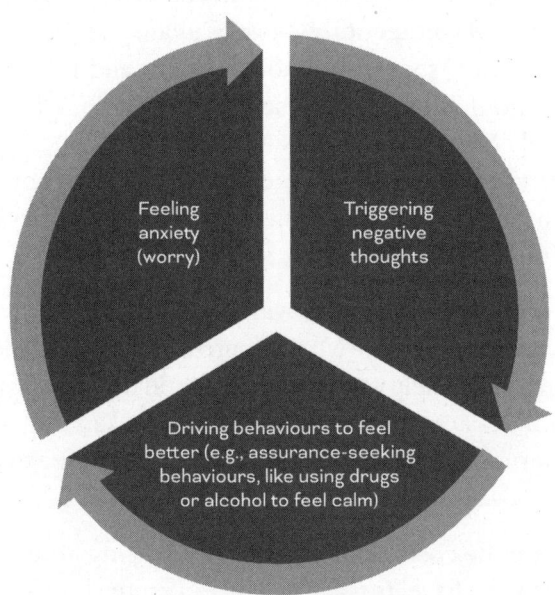

When your persistent worrying increases how threatening you perceive an issue to be, it's common to believe your ability to cope goes down. Prolonged worry can be painful. One way to deal with worry is through exercises designed to challenge it. It's important to write out your answers to help you be objective and evaluate what you're noticing.

This step explores worry by providing ideas to challenge it. The following questions (adapted from Robert Durham) explore the link between worry and feelings of isolation and loneliness.[3]

What are you predicting will happen concerning your future social connections? What is the likelihood it will happen? What do you believe about your ability to build healthy social connections in areas of your life you want, such as work, family, or partnership?

What are your best-case and worst-case scenarios of future social connections? Most of us are good at defining our worst-case scenario. Take a moment and think about yours. Now think about your best-case scenario. What does it look like? What do you believe the chances are that you'll be able to achieve it? To create the social connections you want in your future, you first need to allow yourself to focus on them.

If the worst-case scenario were to happen, what would you do to cope? Explore what resources and coping skills you could tap into to help you cope effectively and be healthy even in a worst-case scenario. Worry can be unlocked with a plan and internal belief that you have the ability or desire to learn how to move forward.

What are the costs and benefits of worrying about this? Worrying can have its place. It can be a motivator to ensure

"Worry affects the circulation, the heart, the glands, the whole nervous system, and profoundly affects heart action."

CHARLES H. MAYO, MD, FOUNDER OF THE MAYO CLINIC

you follow through on a commitment. However, too much worry can freeze you in fear and facilitate a self-fulfilling prophecy. Worry can be draining and self-defeating. Be aware of worry and focus on what you can control through proactive practice to help you break your mental trap.

After you reflect on the above questions on worry, pause and consider the following: On a scale of 1 (low) to 10 (high), how much is worrying a concern for you? If you completed the above section, what was your single most important takeaway?

Step 3: Question Your Automatic Negative Thoughts

From a CBA point of view, if you are open to the possibility that your automatic thinking limits your beliefs about your potential, you allow your conscious mind to consider alternatives. When not managed, negative thoughts can lead to catastrophizing (e.g., because someone is five minutes late, your meeting will be ruined). This pattern of thinking leads to misassumptions and increases the risk of jumping to the worst-case situation and, if allowed to run, can generate a self-fulfilling prophecy.

Though isolation and loneliness are not classified as a mental illness by the *Diagnostic and Statistical Manual of Mental Disorders* (DSM-5), the longer a person is experiencing isolation and loneliness, the greater their risk of developing a mental illness like depression or anxiety, or compensation addictions such as drug and alcohol use, work, shopping, sex, and internet overuse.

Whether your thoughts are good or bad, what you focus on and believe influences your view of yourself and the world. Accepting that your negative automatic thoughts could be untrue is helpful because this creates an opportunity to discover the benefits of cognitive restructuring.

> **Check-in**
>
> Do you believe that any of your negative automatic thoughts could be misguided?
>
> If yes, how so? If no, what evidence would you need to be convinced they're wrong?

When you discover that negative thoughts can be wrong, you set the stage to learn how to release their power over you. The benefit of practicing cognitive reframing is that it can teach you how to free yourself from self-judgement, self-loathing, and other self-attacks associated with automatic negative thoughts.

Since automatic negative thoughts come without invitation, it's helpful to learn how to uninvite them and let them go or reframe them.

Positive thoughts come from engaging in healthy activities you enjoy and being around people you trust and enjoy, and happiness is the natural state you enter when you're not distracted by negative thoughts and emotions.

I didn't get this until I noticed that when I'm walking my dog, Dozer, my mind shifts from the business of the world to watching him sniff in excitement as he discovers who was on the trail before us. After the combination of watching Dozer moving, the fresh air, the vistas, and my mental state, I can't recall ever coming back to the car after a walk not feeling good inside. I leave my cellphone in my car to ensure I don't get distracted on these 45-minute walks down the abandoned railway track.

The more you learn how to teach your mind to focus on positive thinking and engage in activities that you enjoy, the more likely you'll be able to unlock your mental trap.

8

Unlocking the Mental Trap

IF YOU'VE STARTED to practice your daily resiliency microskills exercises—such as journaling, mood tracking, and cognitive reframing—you may be noticing you've loosened or even unlocked your mental trap. In your journal, you can track how your work is positively impacting your thinking, emotions, and behaviour. Learning to challenge negative thoughts is a skill. Once you learn the skill, you can apply it to all areas of your life, so that you can feel confident engaging in social connections that can lead to authentic relationships.

Your mind is constantly wandering—about 47 percent of the time, regardless of what you're doing.[1] Humans are the only species on the planet that can plan for tomorrow while thinking about yesterday. Because there's so much going on in our mind as it's jumping around, we can feel overwhelmed and mentally tired. Our default mode network, which is constantly generating thoughts, can be slowed down by mindfulness and meditation.[2] I've introduced resiliency skills like the three-minute meditation so that you can learn mind control: being able to slow your mind from jumping around. In a calmer mind state, you can engage in the activities in this chapter, which take on the negative thinking that creates mental traps.

What I know from supporting people as they learn how to take control of their thinking is it requires conviction and motivation. Much like learning how to ride a bike, you must persevere after a fall and continue the process of learning.

I had the opportunity to watch each of my three children learn how to ride a bike. Each had their share of spills. After they fell and I addressed their bumps, scratches, or cuts, and comforted them through their pain and tears, I don't recall ever having to encourage them to keep on trying. They would just ask me to help them try again. They wanted to win. Their victory was learning how to ride their bike. They got back on their bikes because the perceived reward was greater than the fear of falling. Thirst for something we want and value is a powerful motivator.

To move away from isolation and loneliness requires the same conviction. Committing to learn and practice these cognitive-behavioural approach (CBA) concepts can help you unlock your mental trap. And unlocking your mental trap permits you to begin to make new social connections.

Practice Skills That Can Remove Negative Thoughts and Emotions

Shakespeare's Hamlet said, "There is nothing either good or bad, but thinking makes it so." History gives us examples of many who have significantly changed themselves and helped change others' lives through what they believed to be true.

Mental traps form because of self-destructive thinking.[3] Typically, self-defeating thinking can put individuals at risk of engaging in self-destructive behaviours. The mental trap's negative beliefs can take an emotional toll on an individual's experience.

Viktor Frankl's survival of a Nazi death camp contradicts the widespread attitude that the environment controls an individual's happiness. Frankl didn't accept the notion that his destructive reality controlled his ability to be happy and find peace. He demonstrated to the world that the power of choice and freedom can't be taken from us as long as we choose not to let it. He not only survived the camp, but he also grew spiritually and intellectually. His amazing journey is a reminder that we all have a choice of what we want to think, regardless of the situation. William Glasser agreed with Frankl that we have choice over how we view the world and how we deal with our difficulties, regardless of how we have been taught to respond.[4] Glasser's point is we all can learn new and better ways to think.

How Do You View the World?

If you tend to catastrophize—that is, you make strongly negative interpretations about minor life setbacks—this will strengthen your mental trap. We feel and do as we think, and we feel good when we think straight.[5] At any given point in your life, your thoughts, feelings, and behaviours reflect how you cope under pressure.

Personality is how we interact and filter the world. Building on cognitive schemas and cognitive distortions, if you don't learn how to challenge your automatic negative thinking, you risk feeling trapped. The path away from isolation and loneliness runs between your ears.

Edmund J. Bourne provides examples of four lenses that describe how we view and interact with our world:[6]

Worrier: The worrier creates anxiety by imagining the worst-case scenario. Their typical reaction to any physical ailment is panic. They anticipate the worst, always catastrophizing and looking for symptoms or signs of trouble. Their favourite expression is "what if." This type promotes unbearable anxiety, resulting in avoidance behaviour. They also become anxious about anxiety.

Critic: The critic is on constant alert, judging and evaluating. They always expect failure, put themselves down, or make themselves dependent on others. The critic emphasizes weakness and inadequacies, negatively labelling everything that happens around them. Their favourite expression is "I'm stupid." Consequently, their self-esteem is low.

Victim: The victim feels hopeless and helpless, believing that there's something wrong and obstacles are insurmountable. Their favourite expression is "I can't." This kind of thinking results in depression.

Perfectionist: The perfectionist is similar to a critic. Instead of putting themselves down, they push forward constantly, telling themselves that their efforts are not good enough and that they should be working harder. Always looking for external validation of their self-worth, their favourite expression is "I should." Chronic stress and burnout mark this thinking.

Take a moment and evaluate your own personality tendencies. You might identify with one type more than another, or you might be a combo, like a Worrier-Perfectionist.

How to Challenge Irrational Beliefs

Negative beliefs might be "should" or "must" statements, or they can be words, images, mental pictures, or memories. Some of them come from your proven beliefs or from events that lead you to form self-statements. These statements represent the conclusions you've drawn from the faulty data you have from unchallenged irrational beliefs. To identify irrational thoughts and beliefs, notice what goes through your mind when you're having a strong feeling or a strong reaction.

When you detect an irrational belief, dispute it. Disputing can be cognitive, emotive, or behavioural. In this stage, you focus on evidence, data, information, and facts, not on your interpretation of events or situations. You're looking for information that supports or doesn't support your irrational thoughts. This will help you clarify your thinking and reduce the intensity of distressing feelings.

Dispute the evidence: Ask, "Where does it say I need to be perfect? Show me the evidence."

Learn the predictable outcome: Ask, "What will happen if I continue to act this way?"

Play with the irrational thought: Ask, "If I continue to believe I need to be Superman, what will I gain from it?"

The act of looking for evidence requires you to be specific about the facts. Doing some mental research to find unfounded or unproven opinions is necessary. The following examples are some questions you may use in disputing your irrational thinking. Choose the most applicable to your thinking problem.[7]

- What is the evidence for this belief?
- Looking objectively at all my life experiences, what is the evidence that this is true?
- Does this belief invariably or always hold true for me?
- Does this belief promote my well-being?
- Did I choose this belief on my own, or did it develop out of my experience of growing up in my family?
- Have I had any experiences that show that this thought is not always completely true?
- When I'm not feeling this way, do I think about this type of situation any differently? How?
- When I felt this way in the past, what did I think about that helped me feel better?
- Have I been in this situation before? What happened? Is there anything different between this situation and previous ones? What have I learned from prior experiences that could help me now?
- If I look back at this situation five years from now, could I view it any differently?

Unlocking your mental trap will require you to learn how to control unwanted negative thoughts. As we move into Part III, our focus will be closing social connections gaps. Keep in mind that it's normal to slip back to old thinking when stress is intense. Use resiliency techniques such as deep breathing to find calm and then practice your CBA skills to help regain your composure. As with any new skill, making it a habit requires time, practice, and patience.

If you put into practice the information presented in this chapter, you'll position yourself to reap the rewards and benefits of being more in control of your thinking, feeling, and behaving. Knowing that you oversee how you think, what you do, and how you feel is an excellent starting point to unlocking your mental trap.

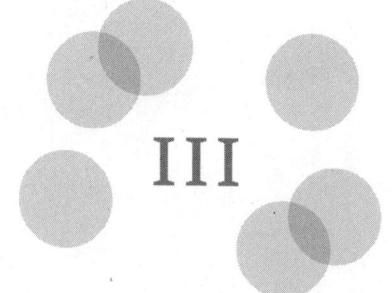

III

How to Build Authentic Connections

9

The Path to Authentic Connections

MY COUNSELLING EXPERIENCE has taught me that each person moves at their own speed. If you feel confident at this point to begin to close social connections gaps, this is indeed good news. You don't need to have your mental trap completely unlocked to begin. Engaging in low-risk social connections activities can help boost your resiliency and mental health.

As you become more mindful and a practiced observer of negative thoughts, you'll reduce the risk of them impacting your mental health. The purpose of this chapter is to prepare you to close social connections gaps through repairing or developing relationships that can become authentic connections.

Mindfulness expert Jon Kabat-Zinn teaches that self-healing power comes from self-awareness by simply paying attention to your purpose in the present moment.[1] Once you've decided you want to close social connections gaps, you're in position to become more aware of how your day-to-day actions play an important role in achieving this outcome. If for any reason you experience fear or anxiety as you begin this process, don't become discouraged. By being non-judgemental and patient, and continuing to practice your resiliency and cognitive-behavioural approach (CBA) skills, you can reset.

You now know that negative thoughts happen and you can be mindful of them, without reacting to them. If they want to hang around, that's fine; if they want to leave, that's fine as well. No one is perfect. There's no way to stop negative thoughts from happening. But you do know that you have a choice as to how you'll deal with them.

Self-Compassion

As you learn to unlock your mental trap, you can also begin to develop an authentic connection with yourself. Much like a calm mind, a kind mind is also a happy mind.

Self-compassion is helpful as you take on the challenge of closing social connections gaps. Self-compassion is like supporting someone you care about through a difficult time and the person you're supporting is yourself. Self-compassion begins with acknowledging that when you fail, it's hard and difficult and it's a part of learning. Being kind to yourself can provide you with the space to learn and grow, one experience at a time.

Practice self-kindness: Treat yourself the same as you would treat a beloved child, friend, family member, or pet who fails, by displaying empathy, tolerance, and patience and by encouraging yourself to try again. When self-criticism and self-loathing are active, ask how these thoughts help you feel better. Self-kindness is about accepting the situation, identifying what you can control, and preparing to move forward by focusing on what you want, not on what you don't have.

Be mindful of emotions: Self-compassion can be facilitated by accepting some wisdom from Eastern thinking—that our automatic negative thoughts are nothing more than thoughts. They're just random information, and there's no evidence that they're true or hold any divine truth. When you don't overidentify with negative thoughts, which lead to negative feelings, you allow them to leave as fast as they arrive.

Authentic Relationships Fundamentals

All authentic relationships have two core principles: psychologically safe interactions and a desire by both parties. A one-way relationship where you want someone's friendship is not enough: the other party must want what you want. Many people become isolated or lonely after they often have been hurt or experienced some rejection. Or they failed to develop or maintain a relationship that meets their need for social connection.

Authentic connections are positive social interactions that create good feelings and are perceived as being positive by both parties. Authentic relationships are congruent; you can't fake them. Humans are good at picking up when someone is being real. Once you stop believing another person's intentions are genuine, it's unlikely you'll want to continue trying to build an authentic relationship with them.

Maintaining an authentic relationship requires effort, desire, and intention. Authentic relationships are like a car: to keep them working optimally, you must pay attention to warning signs, do your checkups, and make repairs when needed. An example of authentic relationship repair is if you do something wrong or make a mistake, you apologize, take responsibility, and are willing to fix it. One way to check if you're in a truly authentic connection is by measuring the degree of motivation you have to show up and be present. For the most part, authentic relationships are easy to maintain; they feel good and often charge your battery.

Most relationships have tough patches. However, as long as both parties are motivated to work through their challenges, and are willing to take responsibility for their actions, things typically can be worked out.

The path to discovering and building new authentic connections is not about being lucky, though some good luck here and there can't hurt. Most of the time, it ultimately comes down to setting personal goals concerning social connections.

As you do so, it's important to be mindful of your expectations. People who experience isolation and loneliness can set unrealistic expectations for themselves and others. Pay attention to your expectations, and test them through conversations as soon as you can to get feedback on what's realistic and what may be unrealistic.

Accept that to close social connections gaps you'll need to be open to taking risks. The antidote for isolation and loneliness is authentic social connections, which require interacting and getting along with other people who will have different wants and expectations. Not all social connections will become authentic connections. The good news about being human is that even micro-social connections—such as saying hello at the coffee shop to the clerk who serves you each day—are good for your mental health.

Though positive social connections can be exceptionally good for mental health, negative social connections can be equally bad. As you begin the process of building or rekindling authentic connections, it's helpful to be clear on what an authentic connection is. Let's pause to revisit what an authentic connection is and what it's not.

"The meeting of two personalities is like the contact of two chemical substances: if there is any reaction, both are transformed."

CARL JUNG

> **Check-in**
>
> - What are five things that would tell you you're in a positive authentic connection?
>
> - What are five things that would tell you you're not in an authentic connection?

Below are some qualities of authentic and inauthentic connections. Understand that any negative factor may be enough to flag a relationship as not authentic. The more negative factors, the more likely the relationship is not genuine and there's some risk in continuing the relationship if the concerns are not resolved. Perhaps one of the hardest things to do when we feel isolated, lonely, and crave acceptance and social connections is to set boundaries around what we will and will not tolerate.

In an authentic connection, the two people:

- Care for each other's best interests

- Trust each other

- Are willing to support each other

- Communicate well with each other

- Resolve conflict in a positive manner

- Engage in a psychologically safe relationship and feel psychologically safe when interacting

- Equally value and want the relationship

- Are open and honest with each other
- Value their social connection
- Feel good after interacting with each other
- Have a positive outlook on their work and life, and are willing to support each other through challenges
- Have the same interest level in the other's needs and wants

Signs that a connection may not be authentic include:

- One or both don't follow through on commitments
- Anger and argument are constant
- No expression of kindness
- One person does things for the other person with no reciprocation
- One or both don't trust each other
- One or both fear the other's behaviour (e.g., anger)
- One or both are constantly disappointed
- One or both don't appear to benefit from the relationship
- One or both regret having to spend time together
- One or both constantly lie
- One or both are constantly negative about life, work, and the world
- One or both have different expectations around needs and wants
- One or both don't feel psychologically safe when interacting

Setting Boundaries

Personal boundaries represent the behaviours you won't tolerate under any circumstances. Oprah Winfrey, one of my heroes who I think has done so much to help us all look closely at ourselves, provides some clear examples of personal boundaries, which I've paraphrased here:[2]

- Don't go through my personal belongings
- Don't criticize me
- Don't make comments about my weight
- Don't take your anger out on me
- Don't humiliate me in front of others
- Don't tell off-colour jokes in my company
- Don't invade my personal space

It's helpful to write out your boundaries: the minimum you won't tolerate. To do so, answer this question, "What will I not tolerate in a personal relationship under any circumstances?" This can be a hard question to answer when you want to be accepted and no longer want to feel alone. However, if you don't identify your boundaries, you may be trading in one problem for an entire set of different problems. Let me share my thoughts on my own personal boundaries as an example:

- I'm a watcher and pay attention to what people take and not return. I naturally like doing things for people I care about. However, I've learned that people can get used to taking and not giving back.

- I do what I say I'll do, and I watch closely how much a person follows through with what they say they'll do. Respect is important to me; not following through is a sign of disrespect.

- I don't like pushing myself on others if they don't want to accept me. I often fade away quietly. I stop trying.

- I'm clear of my personal boundaries and how they were formed. They come from my childhood, around being adopted.

- Trust is a complex issue for me, and at my age I'm not sure if it will get any better. My mental trap is the constant management of fear of rejection.

I share this because no matter how we present ourselves to the outside world, we have a private world that influences our thinking, feeling, and behaviour. No one wants to be alone, and it's important to feel welcomed, wanted, understood, and safe in all authentic relationships. It's also important not to compromise your values or personal boundaries. When you don't feel the other person cares as you do, then you're likely not in an authentic relationship. I say that because if you're in an authentic relationship—especially an intimate relationship—your partner will want to understand how to close any gaps and remove any fears or concerns about their level of commitment. Relationships can be complex and hard because of emotions. More importantly, they're two-way, and while they don't have to be perfect, they must be honest, transparent, and equal.

> **Check-in**
>
> List three items on your personal boundary list—things you will not tolerate, like lying, cheating, or physical abuse.

If any of your social connections is toxic or exhibits negative behaviour, such as the traits outlined above, consider how to fix or end the relationship. Because if you don't, such a relationship can drain your energy and prevent you from finding healthier social connections. Though you can't choose your family, you can choose how you'll interact with them and set boundaries for what you'll tolerate from them.

> **Stay safe**
>
> Many people may never believe they could find themselves in a violent domestic situation or involved with a criminal. If you ever realize you're in such a situation, understand that there's help available; you're not alone.
>
> Call a local mental health resource, crisis line, or 911. Explain your situation and ask for guidance. You don't have to figure this out alone, and you don't have to be in danger.

Authentic Connections Inventory

Regardless of your current situation, you likely have had some experience with authentic relationships in your life. You may have some in place today, people with whom you can engage in different situations, such as work or community. If you don't think you've ever had an authentic relationship, even for a short time, please read on, as you may discover you've had some experiences but have forgotten them.

Authentic relationships have different levels of intensity that come with different levels of expectations. The most intense relationships are with a partner; the least intense with someone you've just met. For each of the five levels, fill in the names of the people in your life today with whom you are in an authentic relationship.

- **Level 5—Intimate:** partner relationship that involves commitment, love, and sex
- **Level 4—Valued:** children, other family members, and friends who are highly valued and often loved
- **Level 3—Trusted:** close friends or colleagues with whom there is a mutual level of respect and caring for well-being
- **Level 2—Intermittent:** a liked person where interactions are unplanned or irregular; share common interests, history, experience, and respect for each other
- **Level 1—New:** a person just met and felt a connection; have agreed to follow up and to keep your conversation going

Authentic relationships can evolve or decline. For instance, someone was in Level 3 for years and then the relationship evolved to Level 4 and shortly after to Level 5. The opposite can happen, where a Level 5 relationship lessens to Level 3 or the relationship ends.

Authentic Connection Areas

There are different areas of your life where you can build authentic connections, such as:

- **Work:** people you work with (e.g., clients and colleagues)
- **Community:** people you interact with at local gyms, clubs, and other community spaces or events

- **Friendship:** people you associate with to foster personal bonds and supportive relationships
- **Family:** children, parents, cousins, in-laws, and extended family

For many people, their social connections at work and in the community are important for fulfilling social connections. Though most people want an authentic connection with a partner (a Level 5 relationship), as there are positive benefits for our long-term health and happiness, we also benefit from having many other kinds of authentic connections.

Authentic Connections Regret

As you review your current authentic connections, what may pop into your head is regret over some you may have lost. The reasons for the lost connection can vary, from a falling-out, death, change of life circumstances, or a move. The good news is if the person is still alive, you can explore ways to move past regret and rekindle the relationship. We sometimes just stop working at a relationship and it loses its spark and connection. Mental traps can create cognitive dissonance (e.g., "They're not that important to me"), to rationalize why not to reach out. As you unlock your mental trap, if there are relationships you have some regret losing and would like to mend or revisit, make a note of them. When you're ready, you can try to rekindle them, keeping in mind that it takes two to have an authentic connection.

> **Check-in**
>
> Is there anyone with whom you've lost touch and would like to reconnect?
>
> Write down the following for each lost connection you would consider reconnecting with: name, the reason you lost touch, estimated time of last contact, and what you think it would take to rekindle it (e.g., apology, call).

Relationship Management 101

Why a previously authentic connection no longer exists may not matter as much as your intention to reconnect. The outcome is out of your control; you can only control your behaviour. However, some basic relationship management may help get things back on track.

- Be open to talking and listening to each other without judgement.
- Release all negative thoughts and emotions.
- Take responsibility for your actions.
- Provide an opportunity for both sides to share what they'd like to see stopped or started.
- Be collaborative to find a resolution that works for both sides.
- Create a plan if further action is needed.
- Apologize when appropriate.

"To build authentic relationships you need to lead with generosity and serve them first."

KEITH FERRAZZI

- Follow through on agreements.
- Forgive but don't forget. If you're struggling with forgiveness, explore The Forgiveness Project.[3] You may be inspired by some of the stories and benefits for people who've learned to forgive. Carrying around a negative anchor of regret can be hard on your mental health and view of the world.

Knowing the value of authentic connections—they charge your resiliency batteries and support your mental health—can help motivate you to maintain them in the tough times.

An old negative thought ("I don't care about them or need them") that pops into your head because of a challenging moment can fire off an old script that allows old beliefs to slip back into your head, changing your mental state and mood. Be mindful that the mental trap, as quickly as it became unlocked, can lock you up again in a negative state. Keep practicing your resiliency exercises, so you have the reserves to move through challenging moments.

Understanding the mental trap in these moments is extremely helpful, as it can give you a moment to calm down and regain your composure. With a clearer mind, you can focus on what you want. Most times, we don't want to lose an authentic relationship, but if the mental trap is in charge, it can create confusion, turn small issues into bigger ones, or inhibit the desire and motivation to fix an interpersonal conflict.

During these stressful times, be careful not to apply "Band-Aid solutions," such as going out and buying a gift, expecting it will fix the problem. More times than not it will only lead to more disappointment. Things don't fix conflict; people talking honestly and openly does. Finding a solution requires that both parties want the relationship and are willing to fix the issue.

Authentic relationships adhere to the law of reciprocation, which means they are give and take. For example, you offer an act of kindness, like inviting someone to dinner at your home. In an authentic relationship, the person you invite would want to reciprocate in some way. If they don't and are just taking advantage of your kindness, you won't be motivated to continue the relationship. Keep in mind that it takes two to have a relationship, and you can't force people to do things they don't want to.

Take Jack and Jill, for example. They connect super-fast, bonding at their first meeting. Both single and tired of the dating scene, they are both seeking a serious relationship—a long-term, authentic relationship. Jack is an introvert; Jill, an extrovert. Jill wants to chat with Jack several times a day. Jack has positive feelings for Jill but finds her expectations to chat several times a day mentally exhausting.

It's a critical point for Jack to share his concern. If he's fearful that being honest may hurt Jill, his incongruency can create resentment and frustration at trying to keep up to Jill's expectations. He may reach the point that he just can't do it anymore and break up with Jill for a reason Jill may never understand. If Jack can feel confident and safe to tell Jill the truth, that he enjoys his time with her but is finding the expectation to communicate many times a day too much for him, he can set a boundary. He would prefer to communicate once a day, but of course, if there's an emergency he's open to talking any time.

Jill can react in one of two ways. She can be open to working with Jack to find a compromise or get offended and shut down.

For authentic connections to build and last, they require the communication pipes to be kept clean. That requires honest, open, and sometimes difficult conversations to ensure both parties feel congruent and connected. Relationships are emotional. If Jack's and Jill's perspectives are not aligned, their authentic connection can end quickly.

Free Choice Is a Free Choice

One of the hardest and most rewarding things you'll do in life is maintain all your authentic relationships: it requires energy, time, commitment, and intention. Much like a garden, you need to keep tending to them and address the weeds as they pop up.

At the core of why relationships can be difficult emotionally is free choice. You have the right to decide who you want to build an authentic relationship with. It's your right as well as the other person's. Authentic relationships don't come out of any trickery, bribing, begging, or any other silly thing humans do to try to get someone to like us. They're simply the evolution of two people who find a connection that both value and find beneficial. You'll often be attracted to people with whom you have common interests, passions, purpose, values, and visions, and who demonstrate an interest in who you are.

Managing your mental trap is important when someone doesn't show interest in you after you have shown interest in them. Discovering new authentic relationships is like mining: you won't always dig up gold. What's important to keep in mind when someone doesn't show interest in you is that they may have something else they're dealing with that you're not aware of. Or maybe it is you. Regardless, it doesn't matter if you try to get to know someone and they reject you; that's a part of the deal because of free choice. Just because you want something doesn't mean you'll get it—especially an authentic relationship. Why? You guessed it: because it takes two people who want the same thing.

At its core, building authentic connections is dependent on free will and accepting that not every person will want to get to know you, nor will you want to get to know every person. Engaging in social activity enables you to meet new people. From there, you both decide the next steps.

Thomas Edison, who invented the light bulb, didn't look at all his failed attempts as failures. He reframed his failures as learning opportunities that got him one step closer to his desired outcome. When you are open to learning from rejection, like Edison, you may get a few insights from each failure: you tried too hard; you didn't follow up; you talked too much; you had a different set of values... None of which is a bad thing, because in the end the person you build an authentic connection with needs to accept the real you. "You must be you; no one else will do" is a phrase I've said to many clients struggling with rejections. You can't change who you are to impress another person. They'll eventually figure out who you are, and that will only bring future disappointment and heartbreak. It's important to always be who you are.

Of course, if you have some behaviours, such as anger control issues, that are challenging, it's helpful to get these taken care of for your mental health, as they can certainly be barriers. We all can benefit from personal development. The key point is to accept and understand you are you, and the people you want in your life must be okay with the real you. You must be okay with you, too. No human being is perfect. That's a fact. In the end, does it matter why someone rejects you? What matters is for you to understand that through failure comes learning, and there's no other path to successful authentic relationships.

Before you seek authentic relationships, put in place mental protections by setting realistic expectations. Accept that there will be challenges before you reach your goal. Discovering and building authentic relationships requires that you not only understand but also accept that rejection can happen.

Authentic Connection Killers

As you prepare to move away from isolation and loneliness to find new authentic connections, it's of value to be aware of and avoid authentic connection killers:

- **Jealousy:** worrying or accusing a person of engaging in hurtful behaviour
- **Anger:** the feeling of anger is not an issue; it's what a person does when angry that's the issue
- **Control:** attempting to control or manipulate someone
- **Lying:** not being truthful about intentions or actions
- **Shame:** attempting to use guilt or shame to get what you want
- **Lack of follow-through:** not honouring promises

  Authentic connection killers erode trust and respect.

Prepare Yourself to Discover and Build Authentic Relationships

To move from point A (where you are today) to point B (new authentic relationships) requires intention and action. The following 26 tips are meant to provide ideas for your consideration.

- **Be open to yourself first:** Practice self-compassion and develop self-acceptance. Practice positive self-talk. The more you like yourself, the better. People are attracted to people who humbly like who they are. You'll need to be open to learn how to develop an authentic connection with yourself.

- **Prepare for setbacks:** Rejection can and likely will happen. When old thoughts slip in, use the skills you've developed to unlock your mental trap to get you settled and calm. Be mindful and aware that if a tough moment comes along it too shall pass, provided you're letting go of negative thoughts.

- **Keep updating your authentic connections inventory:** As you build new relationships and reconnect old ones, it helps to be mindful of your authentic connections so when you feel isolated or lonely, you know who you can reach out to for support. It's helpful to have evidence in front of you of the people who care for you. All you need to do is reach out.

- **Name your number-one authentic connections gap:** The more authentic connections you have, the better your mental health, and the more you'll feel supported. All connections are beneficial; however, if you feel you're missing one kind of authentic relationship, it's helpful to name it. When you're ready, you can close this social connections gap. If it's an intimate relationship you're seeking, it's helpful to ensure you have a healthy relationship with yourself. Start getting out and meeting people. Focus on the process, rather than the outcome, to take some pressure off yourself. The point is to be clear of what your gap is without hyper-focusing on it.

- **Authentic relationships happen:** You can't make people like you; authentic connections just happen. They can't be forced. The more people you meet and interact with, the more likely you'll make authentic connections.

- **Engage in social activities:** Consider picking one activity to engage in on a daily or weekly basis that has the potential of regular and frequent social connections. Focus on enjoying the activity.

- **Focus on personal connections first:** If you're looking to find an intimate authentic relationship, focus on developing a healthy personal relationship first. Be mindful that an intimate, authentic relationship requires time—typically up to two years—before both parties fully commit to being partners. Become good friends first; allow love to form over time. You can't rush love!

- **Build an inventory of potential activities you could participate in:** Become a volunteer, attend church, join a choir, become active as a coach, take a course, join a local community group like Lions, join a professional group like Chamber, start a hobby, join a club, become a member of a gym, take cooking lessons, engage in social activities.

- **Practice self-compassion:** Accept that your situation is based on your expectations, perceptions, and experiences. What you do with each of these will ultimately be what you think about yourself. Be kind to yourself.

- **Leverage your loneliness drive:** With loneliness often come energy and drive to move away from it. Be aware that this drive can lead to work addiction or other behaviours to escape emotional pain. You can learn how to harness this loneliness drive to make better decisions, such as building a plan to form authentic relationships.

- **End old relationships to build new:** If you're in a relationship that's not authentic and is hurtful, you need to evaluate the risk and potential harm. A toxic relationship can drain your energy or ability to find and build a new healthy one.

- **Expand your frame of reference:** Consider the Buddhist idea of dukkha: accepting that we're all imperfect, and there's no permanence (things change, we get old, we die). There's no escaping the fact that with life comes suffering. Accept that you have a choice to learn how you deal with suffering, and that good times will be followed by bad times, then good times. Nothing is perfect or forever.

- **People need people:** We all need meaningful relationships that are aligned to our values for us to experience happiness. This means there are lots of people out there like you who are looking to build safe and meaningful social connections.

- **Facilitate authentic relationships:** There are things—I call them human gifts—you can do to facilitate relationships, such as showing gratitude to others for what they do; being thankful and authentically appreciating others' actions; being aware of critical dates like birthdays and acknowledging them; and being mindful of relationship equity, meaning doing for others what they find helpful and enjoy, not just what you want.

- **Set communication expectations:** As you work to develop an authentic connection, it's helpful early on to discuss the expectations that will meet both parties' needs around communication frequency and what kinds of communication are best for different topics. Don't ever use text to express concerns. Wait to talk them out in person when possible, or use video so you can see the person's non-verbal cues as you listen.

- **Spontaneity is not a bad thing:** When was the last time you randomly showed up to someone's home without calling or texting ahead of time? Putting the human back into human relationships is showing up and saying hello without an agenda. Some people may not like this, so you talk about it and adapt. Others will be grateful you took the time to say hello.

- **Appropriately use dating and hookup apps or dating services:** These tools and services are facilitators. Before you use one, be clear on why, what you want out of it, and how and when you'll use it. They're not quick fixes for building authentic connections. Marketing can create impressions of opportunities, but at the end of the day, you'll need to stay clear that building authentic connections is a process. Temporary, quick fixes seldom fill social connections gaps. My advice is buyer beware. However, there are dating apps that have been around for years, have good reviews, and have facilitated millions of relationships. Do your homework and check reviews before picking an online dating service.

- **Build a social connections practice:** People like to feel welcomed. It doesn't take much to smile, say hello, wave, open a door, say thank you, and be kind to people. All these micro-behaviours can promote social involvement with others. Engaging others, even in low-stakes situations such as saying hello, can build confidence and micro-skills for deeper social connections.

- **Listen and learn:** Be interested in the other person. The more you get to know who they are and focus on them, the more likely they'll care about you and be interested. You don't need to do a lot of self-promotion. Be interested in learning about the other person more than you are in telling them about you.

- **Admit to mistakes:** If you make a mistake, admit it and own it. Be willing to fix your mistakes. People are attracted to people who take accountability for their actions.

- **Tell stories:** Stories can evoke emotion and interest and can increase your connection with others. Stories can influence others to open up and share their own stories.

- **Respond quickly:** Let people know quickly that you got their message. In this fast-paced world, people appreciate when you get back to them quickly with a note saying, "Hi, got your email; I'll get back to you in a day or so with a response." This is a sign of consideration and caring.

- **Consider talking to a mental health professional:** A mental health professional can help you express your fears and concerns about building social connections without feeling judged. They can help you with your mental trap, explore the kinds of micro-skills you may need to practice, and review expectations. Even if you're doing fine and making progress, talking with a mental health person can be a positive experience. You don't always need to be feeling down or broken to benefit from additional support.

- **Consider new opportunities:** Ways you could meet people that you may not have thought of before include taking a painting class, joining a gym, going to a community centre, attending church, and volunteering.

- **Begin building with people you know:** Expand your social connections by reaching out to people you know that you've not chatted with for a while. By using Facebook, you may find an old high school friend you haven't heard from in years. You may be surprised at how pleased old friends are to hear from you. It often can be a positive boost for you and them.

- **Monitor the intensity of your loneliness:** If you're experiencing loneliness, monitor it and track the emotions you feel daily. Journaling will help you process your day, stay objective, and prevent automatic thoughts from causing you unnecessary emotional strain. If you aren't making progress moving away from isolation on your own, ask for some support. It's still possible to move away from loneliness.

Check-in

- Pick three of the above tips that most appeal to you.
- Consider focusing on them and exploring where they can take you.
- An idea can be like a ripple in a pond. It can start small, and the more you focus on it, the more it can expand.

Insight helps prepare you to discover and build authentic connections. There are things you can do mentally, such as keeping your mental trap unlocked, being clear on what you want, and accepting that it will require intention and effort to move away from isolation and loneliness. There are no magic shortcuts. The good news is we're all the same: we need authentic social connections to fulfill our needs. You may find this hard to believe, but there are people out there right now who are looking to meet you and who want to get to know you. We all want to be wanted and needed by others, and the more we accept our vulnerabilities, the more likely we'll be able to put things in perspective. It requires intention and effort to not be alone in this world.

10

Build Authentic Connections with Intention

ONE OF the most effective strategies to better your mental health is to improve the quality of your social connections. Interestingly, just meeting a stranger on a subway and striking up a small conversation can be beneficial for yourself and the person you talk to.[1] The key action for closing social connections gaps is to position yourself to do so. The road to creating authentic connections must go through the traditional landmarks of any new relationship. The exercises in this chapter are designed to support you to frame the kinds of social connections you want to form.

Sonja Lyubomirsky's research suggests that 50 percent of happiness is genetic, 10 percent is the environment, and 40 percent is what you choose to do with intention.[2] This suggests that a lot of happiness depends on your actions. Moving away from isolation and loneliness requires a decision and conviction.

According to positive psychology research, most of us expect that more of a thing will make us happier. While many people believe that a higher salary has a positive impact on well-being, Daniel Kahneman and Angus Deaton reported that with income levels over US$75,000 a year there was no further well-being benefit.[3] This suggests that money really can't buy happiness; it can, though, impact financial security.

Hedonic adaptation is a theory that suggests human beings will return to their baseline level of happiness, regardless of what happens to them.[4] For example, you fall in love and feel over the moon. This theory says that in time, as you get used to the relationship, it will lose its newness and you'll slip back to your happiness set-point level. The hedonic adaptation treadmill suggests that whatever the positive or negative experience, over time human beings adapt and get used to it as their norm.[5]

This can be a challenge for a person experiencing social connections gaps, isolation, and loneliness because they risk getting used to being uncomfortable. To move forward will require deciding that they want to have more happiness in their life, and recognizing that filling social connections gaps promotes happiness. Keep in mind the benefits of this: happy people's life expectancy is much longer than people who perceive they are lonely.

There's some interesting research estimating the value of social connections in US dollars:[6]

- Volunteer at least once a week; the increase to your happiness is like moving from a yearly income of $20,000 to $75,000.

- Interact with a trusted friend most days; it's like earning $100,000 more each year.

- Visiting trusted neighbours regularly feels like $60,000 a year more.

- A broken social connection, such as a divorce, is like suffering a $90,000 per year decrease in your income.

"History has shown us that courage can be contagious and hope can take on a life of its own."

MICHELLE OBAMA

British behavioural economists quantified that adding one new authentic relationship (e.g., new friend) to day-to-day life is worth up to £85,000 (approximately $120,000) a year in terms of life satisfaction for the loneliest 1 percent of adults and up to £15,500 (approximately $22,000) for the average adult.[7]

New social connections can lead to you feeling emotionally rich.

Your Social Connections Experiments, One Step at a Time

The following nine-step model is designed to provide a game plan for taking concrete micro-steps toward discovering and building social connections that can become authentic relationships. This road map moves you step by step with intention, focused on one social connection at a time. As you gain confidence and get results, you'll benefit from increased social connections. You can repeat this model over and over until you've developed all the social connections you want.

You can also use this model to rekindle or repair old relationships. Lessons from restorative justice suggest that one of the most important things humans need is social connections, and often people struggle because they don't have the skills to solve conflict. To repair harm requires nothing more than a willingness to listen, an openness to understand the harm and what it will take to fix it, and the willingness to fix it.

Having a structured action plan with clear goals is critical. In the event that you become frustrated or discouraged, use your action plan to regain your focus, purpose, and motivation. In the world of counselling psychology, we often call plans designed to change behaviour "treatment plans." A treatment plan defines what will be done, when, and what success will look like. The treatment plan is then measured to determine if it's helping the client reduce their mental health symptom load. Because this isn't therapy, you'll call yours an action plan and it will have specific goals and action steps. However, like a treatment plan, it's important to regularly measure if the plan is moving you closer to your desired outcome.

Each of the nine steps has specific questions and activities. Think of this as a plan-do-check-act (PDCA) action plan that you'll develop, adapt, and change, like any continuous improvement model.[8] There's no finish line: once you discover and build authentic relationships, you maintain them, which requires continuous intention.

Success will be dependent on your ability to keep managing your mental trap. Once you engage in the activities and begin to expand your social connections and gain more confidence, this can help keep your mental trap unlocked. You'll notice as you begin to expand your social connections—even by one new connection—that you're on the road to moving away from isolation and loneliness.

Step 1: Establish Your Authentic Connections Baseline

The goal of this journey is to assist you to build authentic connections. We'll begin by getting a baseline of where you perceive you are now. We'll repeat this quick, three-item scale throughout this process to measure your progress. Using the scale of 1 (strongly disagree), 3 (moderately agree), or 5 (strongly agree), rate your degree of confidence for each statement.

- I have authentic connections in my life I'm satisfied with.
- I'm confident I can close my social connections gaps.
- I can keep my mental trap unlocked under pressure.

Total score: ____

The maximum score you can get is 15. The lower your score, the less confident you are. Don't be discouraged if your score is low. This is your baseline. By remeasuring, you can objectively evaluate your progress. One reason why cognitive-behavioural approach (CBA) techniques have been successful is constant measurement. If for any reason you're not getting results, adjust your plan, or consider if your mental trap is challenging you. Practicing resiliency and CBA micro-skills, like you would with physical exercise, can help rewire your brain to achieve the outcomes you want.

Step 2: Imagine Success

Consider what developing authentic connections will look like in your life. Will it mean feeling more confident in your informal interactions, such as smiling at others on the street? Perhaps it means forming meaningful social connections that support your mental health. Keep an eye on your desired outcome while regularly measuring your success on your journey.

Step 3: Tune In to Your Motivation

Why do you want to improve your social connections? Expand your response beyond that you want to feel better. Be thoughtful and finish the following phrase: "Because I want..."

Clarity on your *why* will anchor your vision, and you can draw upon it to stay engaged during any challenging moments. Your *why* provides the link to your inspiration and purpose. Motivation, when defined and intentional, can be the drive to commit to this process. The outcome is positioning yourself to close social connections gaps and to discover and build new authentic connections.

> **Check-in**
>
> - How would you describe your efforts toward building social connections over the past 90 days?
> - How would you describe your results?

The purpose of these questions is to explore what you may already be doing. If you've been trying this process, it can help to add more structure. If you haven't been trying, this process is about getting you to do so.

What are you willing to do to improve your social connections?

Though it may sound like a loaded question, it's not meant to be. I appreciate it can be a difficult one to answer. The word "willing" refers to openness and attitude.

To move away from isolation and loneliness will require you to be willing to do things differently when needed. To close social connections gaps requires that you accept that you need to make some changes.

Step 4: Evaluate the Quality of Your Current Social Connections

The purpose of this step is to now rate the degree of concern you have for each of the five areas: family, partner, friends, work, and community. The area with the highest level of concern may be the area you want to focus on first.

On a scale of 1 (low) to 9 (high), rate your concern about your social connections gaps for each of the following areas of your life. As you do your subjective scoring, it's helpful to consider how you're feeling about each of these areas:

- Family
- Partner
- Friends
- Work
- Community

When you review your results, what is your number-one observation?

Completing an inventory like this one doesn't factor in lost relationships where you may still be experiencing grief or regret. We can't change the past; no amount of worry or angst will change it. What we can do is keep positive memories and focus on them.

Step 5: Determine Your Authentic Connections Focus Area

Using your results from Step 4, decide which area you'd like to focus on first. You certainly can have more than one area; however, let's begin with one to get some traction and prevent you from feeling overwhelmed. By keeping a tight focus, you know where to put your energy. Once you get the success you want, you can expand your focus area.

Once you've picked the focus area you want to start with—family, partner, friends, work, or community—define what you expect the benefit will be for you. Defining success and what a tangible, successful outcome looks like can help you monitor your expectations. Saying you want it because of some feeling (e.g., to feel better) is too vague compared to clarifying a concrete outcome such as "I want a true friend I can be open and talk with, and share my good news and my frustrations."

Now examine what's often called the "so what." This is an expression often used in business when a person is selling an idea to a leader. After the leader listens to the pitch, it's common for them to say, "Okay, so what's the 'so what'?"—meaning "Convince me of the benefit." This helps set expectations and puts a focus on tangible value.

What's your "so what"? What's the purpose of this social connection for you?

Again, something like "to make me happy" could result in frustration and upset. No other person can make you happy. However, different kinds of social connections can fill different needs: a friend can provide companionship; a family can provide a sense of purpose.

List two benefits that you expect fulfilling this social connections focus area will have for you. You don't need to have a perfect answer; you need only have a sense of how you'll benefit from the social connection. It's helpful as you start to pick areas in your life where you'd like to close a social connections gap that you're clear on the benefit. This can help fuel motivation.

Step 6: Prepare for Social Connections Experiments

This preparation step provides a gradual, step-by-step process to help build your confidence to move closer toward what you want: engage in new social connections or rekindle old ones with the potential to become authentic connections.

Exposure therapy teaches that when people avoid something they're fearful of, this could reinforce the fear and make it stronger. This may explain why some people who experience isolation and loneliness become even more withdrawn and fearful of trying. Their fears around trust increase (e.g., "People can't be trusted"). The time we spend unlocking our mental traps creates mental space to be open to trying.

If your mental trap isn't unlocked and fear takes over, it can reinforce negative emotions that confirm the best option is to withdraw and hide from people. Not everyone who experiences loneliness will withdraw; some people have an internal drive to engage in activities that keep them distracted, such as using work to escape loneliness.

Regardless of how you may be coping with isolation and loneliness, the challenge of not having a social connection that meets your needs is still there. Until this is solved, the feelings of isolation and loneliness will continue, because social connections are the antidote to isolation and loneliness. Interestingly, there's no single, agreed-upon term that defines the opposite of loneliness. (I'm not sure "unloneliness" is a word.)

Common fears that stop people from trying to build social connections include fear of failure, fear of people's intentions, and fear of rejection. There certainly can be others. This step introduces a framework, using concepts from exposure therapy, to prepare you to engage in your social connections experiments. Social connections experiments are where you position yourself to interact with others.

As you participate in each social connections experiment, you can teach your brain that there's no real life-threatening danger, so there's nothing to fear. As discussed in an earlier chapter, the fight or flight system is always on to protect you. Having the system going off all the time when you're in no real danger trains your brain to avoid the trigger (e.g., people) that's setting it off. This step can help you retrain your brain to not overreact to triggers so that you can feel calm and in control. With this mental space, you may feel more confident trying to interact with others.

How you retrain your caveman brain is by pairing a situation that triggers fear with a neutral response. This means you can acknowledge the fear and push through it by holding your ground, as you know there's no life-threatening danger. It's this pairing of perceived threat with a neutral response that rewires the brain.

If you recall the guy in the bar example used earlier in this book, if he gets up and says hello to a woman he likes, he learns that the worst that will happen is she won't return the greeting. Through this exposure, if he tried 10 times, he likely would rewire his brain about fear of rejection and discover that saying hello is not painful but a way to meet a new person. Once he removes the fear of rejection, he'll keep trying and eventually meet someone who wants to talk with him.

Through gradual exposure, your brain can learn to dull a trigger so that it doesn't fire off fear. The trick—and what's significant to know about the brain—is it works best when it's warmed up. Like before you sprint as fast as you can, it's in your best interest to warm up so you don't pull a muscle that could keep you from running again until you heal.

When engaging in your social experiments, it's important to know that a little anxiety and fear are good, as this warms your brain and helps to make the new neuro connections needed to teach your brain not to be fearful of the old trigger. Your unconscious brain will learn that for each non-lethal trigger paired with fear, it doesn't need to turn on and instead learns the trigger is neutral—not dangerous but safe. This releases your level of anxiety and fear and will help to keep your mental trap unlocked.

If you start a social connections experiment and don't finish it, that can cause your brain to think you can't overcome this fear, only reinforcing old wiring. Don't worry. You can attempt each step several times.

However, any time you start to struggle in this step, it's helpful to go back and repeat some of your resiliency and CBA micro-skills. Also, as you move through this process, keep in mind the benefit of being mindful: notice how you're doing; focus on the moment.

By successfully taking each step, you're using gradual exposure to overcome targeted fear. One key to success is to focus on micro-steps, one at a time. You can begin to build a fear hierarchy from your least fearful to most fearful actions as they relate to making social connections. Your perception of fear will influence the design from low to high.

Social Connections Experiment

In this example, the targeted goal is to develop one new authentic professional relationship (Level 3 authentic connection). I've included the micro-steps to achieve the goal, and then in italics the realistic expectations—the reason behind the goal.

- Join a professional online community like LinkedIn. *To meet new professionals.*

- Research LinkedIn professionals who have the same interests as you and with whom you could see a potential alignment. *To find like-minded professionals based on their profile.*

- Pick three people you would like to meet. *To focus on who I will try with first.*

- Invite each person to connect to your professional network and explain why you invited them. *To reach out to see if they're interested in connecting; no expectation they'll all want to connect.*

- If they accept, follow up with a thank-you message. *Just because they connect doesn't mean they'll want a professional relationship beyond being a LinkedIn connection.*

- Share posts and follow their activity. Make comments on their posts. *Show some interest in posts I find interesting. This will help me discover alignment and interests.*

- If you find them interesting, enjoy their work, and see common ground, use Messaging to send them a few comments with a specific question. *Reach out for the goal of more formal sharing of professional interests. No expectation a person will respond or be interested but will try. Will only reach out to people I find professionally interested in getting to know better.*

- Wait for their response. If they seem interested, share a few more communications. *No pressure; it's important to allow this to be an organic process. If they're interested, they'll respond.*

- If you're having a two-way communication that appears you both are benefitting from, move to email to continue sharing ideas. *Moving from a LinkedIn conversation to an email conversation is the first step to a more formal professional relationship. It's a positive step.*

- If email exchange is positive, explore an opportunity to talk on the phone to continue to build the relationship. *Continue the process of building trust and credibility.*

- If there are value and interest to move from talking to meeting in person, look to schedule a meeting or to do a video conference. *If the opportunity presents itself and there's a reason to meet in person, or if the person offers, consider the benefits for both parties.*

- If the conversation goes well, continue to follow up and build trust. *Allow the relationship time to evolve. People typically work with people they trust, so this process can take time.*

- Explore an opportunity to work together. *When or if the time presents itself, explore the benefit of working together on a first project.*

- Explore a professional relationship. *Based on how the first project or conversation goes, this will frame for both parties how this professional relationship will mature.*

Notice how this hierarchy moves from least to most challenging and is progressive to provide an opportunity for small successes along the way. As you accomplish these small steps, they can act like gates of confidence. Notice also how this process can help you frame expectations. By going slowly with intention, you can reduce fear and set realistic expectations.

You won't be able to jump from the first step to filling all social connections gaps. Building relationships is a process. The key is to take things slowly and to start with experiments that provoke the least anxiety for you. Once you master this level, move to the next.

Preparing for Your Social Connections Experiment

Using the above example, create your own action plan using the focus area you selected in Step 5. Map out your micro-steps from the least fearful to most fearful action, and alongside each action, note your realistic expectation for it. These micro-steps will help you build confidence and minimize the risk of old thinking and feelings from overwhelming and stopping you on your journey. Lean in to your social connections experiment bit by bit to put each step in your rear-view mirror. Once you have built your fear hierarchy, you're ready to begin.

The structured format described in this step is designed to reduce fear and to help make the process less intimidating, with its framework to move from point A to point B. It's up to you to determine if you'd like to use it.

What's important to keep in mind is how to balance expectations and fear of rejection. Many relationships do not evolve because of misalignment around expectations. It's fine to have boundaries around core values—for example, you may not want to associate with a person who lies to you. However, expecting a person you meet three times to commit to you forever is unrealistic. As you prepare to engage in a social experiment, it's helpful to be clear on your expectations. This is why I like the fear hierarchy: it's focused on one step at a time, and it has realistic expectations.

Step 7: Begin Social Connections Experiments

As you begin your social connections experiments, it's important to be focused and mindful that you are working to remove barriers and reduce feelings of loneliness through intention. It doesn't need to be complicated. However, even simple things can appear hard when you don't have confidence.

Social connections experiments can train your brain that there's no major danger and can position you to build new social connections. Answer this question: "What's the worst thing that could happen if I failed a step trying my social connections experiment?"

Typically, trying doesn't make things worse. Trying and failing puts you one step closer to your goal, but to manage failure you must have perspective. Reasons people typically fail can vary. Some common ones are:

- Unrealistic expectations
- Goals that aren't clearly defined
- Failure to celebrate or recognize small wins
- Misjudging the amount of effort it will take
- Changing the goal during the process (i.e., moving the goalpost)
- Unclear what success looks like
- Unsure of the benefit
- No measurement or frame of reference for progress

You can avoid these pitfalls by being mindful, focusing on your desired outcome, and measuring your progress. As you engage in your social connections experiments, monitor and measure how well they're going. By keeping a daily record, you can note your progress one step at a time as you work toward achieving your desired outcome.

- What was your focus for today?
- What are some reflections from today's social connections experiment?

- How do you feel about today's social connections experiment? Rate the experiment on a scale of 1 to 10—the higher the score, the better you feel.

- How confident were you (on a scale of 1 to 10) during this social experiment?

- How socially connected do you feel today? This is your subjective feeling, on a scale of 1 to 10; the higher your score, the more socially connected you feel.

Step 8: Frame Authentic Connections

Once you meet someone with whom it appears there's an opportunity for this social connection to become a Level 3, 4, or 5 authentic connection, there's more work to be done. Here's a reminder of what these levels mean:

- **Level 5—Intimate:** partner relationship that involves commitment, love, and sex

- **Level 4—Valued:** children, other family members, and friends who are highly valued and often loved

- **Level 3—Trusted:** close friends or colleagues with whom there's a mutual level of respect and caring for well-being

At this stage, ensure you're clear on and understand the social connection etiquette for this relationship: the shared expectations (such as how frequently you'll connect) and the stated intentions of both parties. You'll discover this through listening, observing, and asking clarifying questions. Avoid assumptions. We humans are not good at reading minds. When we guess what someone wants, we're more typically wrong than right.

Ask questions and listen. Discover their values, wants, goals, and beliefs. As you learn, your value system will tell you whether you're enjoying the relationship, as will theirs. Here are some guidelines for building and maintaining authentic relationships.

Build a Relationship with Yourself First

As much as you may want to have meaningful relationships with others, it starts with learning to have a relationship with yourself. As I've mentioned before in this book, when we don't accept who we are, and know what we want and what we need, it's difficult to find happiness with another person. An authentic connection involves encouraging and embracing the other person and feeling comfortable sharing needs and wants. Changing for another person to be liked can become a sore spot and a problem in the future, especially if you don't want to change and are only pretending. Authentic relationships for the long term require being authentic with yourself first.

Discover Your Personality Type

Big Five, a free online tool, lets you examine your personality style based on the five-factor model of personality. It's a set of five broad trait dimensions: extroversion, agreeableness, conscientiousness, neuroticism (sometimes named by its polar opposite, emotional stability), and openness to experience (sometimes named intellect).[9] Knowing your personality traits enhances your ability to understand how you're perceived by others. One interesting attribute of the Big Five is introversion to extroversion: it doesn't have as much to do with whether we like to be with people as much as how we're genetically wired and have learned to compensate to recharge our brain.[10] It's good to be aware of what you are, and when you meet people, what they are, so you know how they'll likely operate and what kind of energy they'll require concerning time. The same holds for yourself. If you're an introvert, you may still enjoy being with people for short periods. However, to charge your battery, you'll benefit from time alone.

Share Expectations Up Front

Share your needs and expectations, and get the other person's reactions. Also, be open: your expectations may need to be adjusted. This process is critical, whether in a friend, family, or partner relationship. It's also helpful to check in on expectations from time to time, as people change, as do their wants and needs. Talk about preferences and expectations that are aligned and appropriate to the relationship you want to develop.

Listen and Learn

A lot can be learned by listening and watching. This happens by asking questions and sharing experiences and stories over time. It will help you learn who the person is, as they learn about you.

Be Aware It's a Process

All new and developing relationships go through a process. It's realistic to expect that in forming a new relationship there will be some disagreements and conflict. This is how expectations and boundaries are often formed. Authentic relationships are the outcome of a process where two people get to learn about and trust each other. That takes time and a willingness to work through issues when they arise. One model I like to reference was designed by Bruce Tuckman for teams but is easily adapted to most new relationships.[11]

Forming phase: Both parties are on their best behaviour: polite, kind, and caring. Typically, both are excited about the new relationship.

Storming phase: Parties start to challenge norms, set expectations, and show frustration and conflict over preferences and wants.

Norming phase: Parties work through differences, align expectations, begin to set common goals, can interact, accept feedback, and are willing to learn how to support each other's needs. A level of authentic commitment and caring is formed.

Performing phase: The relationship has evolved into an authentic connection where both parties benefit and show up for each other. The level of the authentic relationship will define the bond and degree of commitment.

Unless both parties want the relationship to continue, care enough about the other person to work through differences, and align on values, the relationship will never get past the storming phase. This can be caused by a misalignment of expectations or one party's lack of interest in the other person's needs or wants.

Reciprocate

One reason why relationships fail is lack of reciprocation. If you're the only one giving kindness, time, and money to a relationship, it won't last. We value fairness, and if we don't feel the other party is reciprocating a relationship, a feeling of unfairness can lead to a loss of interest and motivation to continue it. The reverse is true, too: if you're just taking and not giving, chances are the relationship will be short-lived.

Time Matters

Building an authentic relationship is a process, and it's best to take your time. Go slow and get to know them on their best and worst days. There's no value in rushing.

Align Values

Both parties must want the same thing, or the relationship won't evolve. You can't make another person value you; they must value you on their own. It's helpful to be clear on your most important values, such as health, family, community, and environment. If you value taking action on climate change and you meet a person who doesn't show any regard for that issue, your relationship opportunity is mitigated if you want to be congruent with your values.

Maintenance Matters

You can't have an authentic relationship unless you have a plan as to how you'll maintain it. This is where clear expectations help, such as how much time you'll spend together or how often you'll check in on each other. What's important is it takes two, and you can't take the attitude that you'll wait for them to reach out to you. It's about two people thinking and caring about each other. That requires intention and motivation on both sides to stay in touch and to keep the authentic connection at the level both parties want.

Seek and Provide Support

One line to put into your memory bank and to regularly ask is "How can I best support you?" Forget about the golden rule; adopt the platinum rule: "Do unto others as they would like done unto them." Ask them what you can do; don't guess or assume.

Ask how you can support: Make a habit of asking how you can provide support in the good and bad times. Being kind, helpful, and so forth sounds obvious, but adhering to the premise of not assuming another's needs is crucial; ask a person how you can best support them.

Ask for support when you need it: When you ask for support, be clear on what kind you need. Accept that a truly authentic connection may deeply care about you but may not have the competency or resources to do what you're asking. For example, I live with a mental health issue, and if I want support from my partner, I can't assume she'll know how to support me in the way I may want. Teaching people how to support you is helpful, so they don't feel uncomfortable. Many people don't understand how to support a person in need or crisis. Because of that, they may avoid trying, which is the worst thing, as we know social connections are critical for our mental health.

In my case, I ask for my partner to emotionally support me in these ways: listening to me when I'm feeling stressed, checking in with me, encouraging me, and spending time with me so I'm not alone with my thoughts. Because my partner is open to providing these supports, when I'm experiencing moments of stress and anxiety, she patiently helps me.

Step 9: Measure Authentic Connections Progress

It's helpful to measure the progress of your social connections experiments, above and beyond the daily experiment logs that you keep. Repeat the authentic connections baseline from Step 1 every month as you proceed with your experiments.

Using a scale of 1 (strongly disagree), 3 (moderately agree), or 5 (strongly agree), rate the degree of confidence you have for each of the following statements.

- I have authentic connections in my life I'm satisfied with.
- I'm confident I can close my social connections gaps.
- I can keep my mental trap unlocked under pressure.

    Total score: ____

"Learn from yesterday, live for today, hope for tomorrow. The important thing is not to stop questioning."

ALBERT EINSTEIN

The maximum score you can get is 15. The lower your score, the less confident you are. Don't get discouraged if your score is low.

By tracking your score monthly, you can monitor how you're proceeding with each of the three statements. The higher your score and the longer you can maintain a high score, the more likely it is that you've closed your social connections gaps and are not currently experiencing isolation and loneliness.

The success of this process depends on your ability to keep your mental trap managed, so old negative thoughts don't disrupt your focus and motivation. It also depends on keeping motivated and focused on building social connections every day. The more social experiments you do, the higher the probability you'll make new social connections or rekindle old ones.

If you slip or have a hard time, it's okay. Be mindful that change can be challenging. Go back to your resiliency and CBA micro-skills and keep practicing. If you become frustrated or anxious, get some professional help to give you the additional support to push through. Moving away from isolation and loneliness is possible. Keep in mind that authentic social connections are the antidote.

We all can close our social connections gaps when we have a frame of reference and the tools to do so. The degree and quality of your social connections will be impacted by your ability to not only discover and build them but also to maintain them. Authentic connections are like a financial investment: the more you put into them and the longer you have them, the greater their value to you and the other person.

Loneliness in the Workplace: A Guide for Employers

THIS LAST CHAPTER is designed for employers and leaders. Think about the last of the four pillars of mental health: environmental factors. The environment of the workspace, whether in an office or at home, can play a critical role in supporting employees' mental health. Leaders, who may have already implemented workplace programs that promote physical health, can play a larger role in supporting mental health through promoting meaningful social connections.

There's ample evidence that gaps in employees' social connections can negatively impact their workplace experience. Lonely workers experience a host of negative health consequences, including:[1]

- Greater risk of cardiovascular disease
- Compromised immunity
- Increased risk of depression
- Shortened lifespan

Loneliness at work can be associated with other terms like alienation and lack of support. At its core, loneliness in the workplace, as in other areas of life, is not necessarily about just being alone or feeling lonely. It's about not having quality relationships that meet a person's needs. In the workplace, a lonely employee can display behaviours such as hostility, negativity, or depressed mood. They may be uncooperative and report a perceived lack of control.[2]

Positive or negative, emotions can spread like the common cold. Emotional contagion is when one person's emotions are transferred consciously or unconsciously to another, impacting their emotional state. An employee who's lonely can influence other employees' thoughts and feelings about isolation and loneliness. We have what are called mirror neurons that copy what others do (e.g., someone smiles at you and without thinking you smile back).[3] Have you ever been around a person who made you feel good because of their energy and humour? This is an example of how one person's emotions can impact another's. The same could be said about negative emotions.

When employees feel socially disconnected, isolated, and lonely in the workplace, it can negatively impact an organization's productivity. Lack of social support can lead to employees feeling mental sluggishness that can impair their productivity, decrease creativity, and hinder decision making.[4] The New Economics Foundation suggests that chronic loneliness has cost employers in the United Kingdom around £2.5 billion a year for factors such as increased health concerns, decreased productivity, and increased staff turnover.[5]

On the flip side, positive social relationships strengthen employee retention and productivity, positively impacting the bottom line.[6] There is a direct link between social connections, mental health, and productivity, perhaps even to the point that Simon Sinek suggests in *The Infinite Game*: that it's helpful when senior leaders have a clearly defined just cause (i.e., a defined goal with a clearly defined purpose) they're committed to and promote it, such as, "To positively impact the employees' experience and employees' mental health."[7]

It's important for employers to understand the benefits of closing social connections gaps for promoting positive mental health. Most employers understand why it's important to stop bullying in the workplace to prevent mental harm, for instance. However, the negative consequences for employees who feel isolated and experience loneliness may not be top of mind.

As an expert in the workforce productivity mental health space, I know first-hand how hard it is to get some leaders to focus on mental health as a strategic priority, even with the following kind of evidence:

- By 2030, it's predicted that mental health problems will be the leading cause of mortality and morbidity globally.[8]

- Untreated mental health problems account for 13 percent of the total global burden of disease.[9]

- It's estimated that one in five Canadians experiences a mental illness or addiction problem.[10] This is a big deal for employers, as the financial costs for disability leave for mental illness are about double that of a leave due to a physical illness.[11]

- The World Health Organization estimates that poor mental health costs the global economy US$1 trillion annually in lost productivity.[12]

- Mental illness is the leading cause of disability in Canada.[13]

Though these kinds of stats provide evidence of the magnitude and negative impact of mental illness, it still can be difficult to make employees' mental health a priority. But there's increasing research on the business case for investing in employees' mental health. One recent study found that employers who developed and implemented a mental health strategy reported a median yearly return on investment in mental health programs of $1.62.[14]

Most leaders know and accept that many chronic diseases (e.g., type 2 diabetes) are preventable and are costing organizations unnecessary dollars in lost time and drug costs. It's also common knowledge that if more employees learned to take better care of their health, they would save organizations significant dollars and improve productivity. The solution doesn't need to be complicated. But the sad truth is many employees value their work and money more than their health. As a result, their health suffers. Employers can offer apps, walking challenges, and incentive programs, but these initiatives don't always work over the long term, unless employees make their health a core value and act on it.

The best way to positively impact employees' mental health is not another program or another policy. It's about talking with employees, helping them feel welcomed and included, and exploring what kinds of behaviours can support mental health in the workplace.

Mental Health and Social Connections

Considering that 80 percent of individuals with psychiatric disabilities report feeling lonely, a proportion that's significantly greater than is reported by members of the general population,[15] it would make sense to be proactive and help employees gain insight into the link between mental health and social connections. This may help reduce stigma and assist employees who are struggling to understand the root cause of isolation and loneliness.

One in five Canadians experiences some degree of a mental health concern every day. That means in an organization of 1,000 employees, on any given day, 200 may have reported to work experiencing a mental health challenge that could have impacted their experience and productivity. Of those 200 (whose mental health challenge may or may not have been diagnosed), potentially 160 could have been struggling not only with a mental illness but also with gaps in social connections, resulting in increased perceived isolation loads and risk of loneliness. This number appears to have increased during the COVID-19 pandemic: according to an Angus Reid Institute report, "Half of Canadians (50%) report a worsening of their mental health, with one-in-ten (10% overall) saying it has worsened 'a lot.'"[16]

What's somewhat challenging about isolation and loneliness is that a person could have such feelings for weeks or months but to onlookers still appear productive in the workplace. However, like a slow leak, if not dealt with, effects will typically show up in other areas of their life over time.

The impact that isolation and loneliness have on society hasn't yet gotten the attention it deserves. One reason is perhaps because neither isolation nor loneliness has any formal medical diagnosis, nor have they been formally linked to any preventive medical screening protocols. The *Diagnostic and Statistical Manual of Mental Disorders* (DSM-5), the bible for psychological diagnosis, doesn't consider isolation or loneliness a mental health condition.

My personal belief, now that I'm focused on the negative impact that gaps in social connections can have on mental health, is this issue will require more formal and medical attention to curb it. Isolation and loneliness should be a concern for all working adults, not just senior leadership. Former US surgeon general Vivek H. Murthy suggested in the *Harvard Business Review* that all organizations should make fostering social connections a strategic priority.[17]

> **Check-in**
>
> Do you believe employers can play a role in facilitating social connections in the workplace?
> If yes, what is one thing you think an employer can do?
> If you're a leader, what are you doing to promote psychological safety in the workplace?

Leadership's Role in Supporting Social Connections

Below are six coaching tips for leaders to practice so they can maximize their ability to build psychologically safe relationships with employees. It is difficult for a leader to influence employees' experience if they have not first built a trusted and safe relationship.

- Demonstrate strong intrapersonal skills (e.g., you manage stress and pressure; you're self-directed and well organized).

- Practice effective interpersonal skills (e.g., oral communications, teamwork, listening).

- Be approachable, willing to help others learn, and eager to coach others.

- Become a leader your employees can trust, through your words and actions.
- Be flexible by adapting well to change and supporting others to move through change.
- Treat all employees fairly and equally and do not play favourites.

By practicing the above, leaders will be more likely to engage in conversations with their employees about how they are doing and be in a position to build a meaningful social connection with them.

How to Boost Psychological Safety in the Workplace

Employers who care about employees' psychological health understand and accept that isolation is as risky as any other psychosocial factor. When any psychosocial factor (e.g., isolation) accumulates as stress, it can strain mental health.

Matthew Lieberman, author of the book *Social*, suggests that the human genetic need to connect is no different than our need for water or food.[18] When this genetic need to feel socially connected is threatened, concerns for survival are triggered. As well, when the brain is not focused on a non-social task, it automatically jumps to preparing how to engage in social connections. One key takeaway from Lieberman's work is when human beings experience social connections gaps, their overall well-being will be negatively impacted.

In the context of the workplace, it's uncomfortable when employees are working remotely, don't feel connected with their peers, or lack at least one person in the workplace they feel psychologically safe to interact with.

"People should be conscious of the large contribution made by anything that gets people together easily in the reduction of loneliness and emotional well-being."

DANIEL KAHNEMAN

The average employee spends about seven working days per year stressed out about a work-related problem instead of coming forward with their concern. This reluctance to speak up and deal with an issue costs an estimated production loss of $7,500 per employee.[19] It's estimated that only 23 percent of Canadian workers would feel comfortable talking to their employer about a psychological health issue.[20]

As a leader, do you have a clear sense as to why employees may not feel safe to come forward with their concerns? Some may not feel the workplace is psychologically safe: they may feel apprehensive that if they express their concerns they will be judged, or that speaking out may impact their job security or status on the team.

Psychological safety means employees feel safe and welcomed when they enter the workplace. It also means that employees feel safe to speak their mind without fear of repercussion. Without this confidence, they risk strain on their mental health.

Employees who don't feel psychologically safe can feel isolated and alone in the workplace. Such isolation can feel like a barrier; they may feel like they're on an island, not socially connected with other employees. Over an extended period, they become increasingly at risk of also experiencing loneliness in the workplace. This can negatively impact their outlook on their work and overall mental health.

It's important for leaders to be aware that even if they check in regularly with their employees, those employees may have unspoken concerns about psychological safety. A leader may not be aware that one or more employees may not trust them. Some may interact in the workplace with the facade that things are okay, but underneath they're experiencing some degree of worry or even fear. Employees who aren't coping well or who are unsure how to self-advocate may not feel psychologically safe.

Be open to the possibility that employees may be having different experiences than you observe. Isolation and loneliness are subjective states, depending on a person's perception of their own experiences.

As an employer or leader, you can help insulate employees from isolation and loneliness in these ways:

- **Talk about psychological safety:** Start the conversation by talking about psychological safety. Make it clear that you understand the importance of social connections and that you don't want anyone feeling isolated or alone.

- **Make social connections a strategic priority:** Employees working remotely and employees working on site will have different needs and expectations. Building a culture of inclusion comes down to all employees feeling psychologically safe and welcomed. Make social connections a strategic imperative with the goal that every employee has at least one safe authentic connection in the workplace. It can improve retention and productivity, and support mental health.

- **Measure employees' risk of isolation:** Explore employees' perceived isolation and loneliness through online tools. My online tool, the Mental Fitness Index (MFI)[21] can assist with assessing employee experience with psychosocial factors, program impact, and psychosocial hazards such as bullying, fatigue, isolation, and productivity. Tools like this are designed to help employers obtain evidence of what's working, employee mental fitness, and workplace experience as well as areas to focus on to reduce mental harm and to promote mental health.

- **Provide training for employees:** Training may include webinars focused on understanding isolation and loneliness, what employees can do, and what the employer is doing. As with mental health, there's a stigma around isolation and loneliness, as well as a lack of understanding about how to close social connections gaps.

- **Leverage social connections technology:** There's an opportunity to leverage technology like Hugr Authentic Connections,[22] a mental health support app, to help employees explore how they can improve their social connections at work and outside of it as a way to build and maintain their social support networks.

Employers and leaders can play an important role in supporting employees to build and maintain psychologically safe relationships in the workplace.

Conclusion

ULTIMATELY, we have many opportunities to have meaningful social connections when we put ourselves in position to do so. Perhaps one of the hardest things we need to do first is to develop a loving and caring relationship with ourselves. When we have self-compassion, a clear understanding of our core values, and a desire to show up for ourselves and others, we are ready to build and maintain social connections that may or may not become authentic connections. Not every relationship will work out, as it takes two parties to want the same outcome.

My intention in writing this book is to provide a road map for people struggling with social connections gaps or who want to help others close their social connections gaps. Closing social connections gaps reduces the risk of being negatively impacted by feelings of isolation and loneliness.

In the end, your life will be defined by what you choose to do. You can only control your own actions. Though it can be difficult, one of the most glorious things about being a human is having meaningful social connections. It's worth the effort.

Acknowledgements

I'D LIKE TO acknowledge the wonderful team at Page Two for their amazing partnership, especially Amanda Lewis for your incredible support in helping this dyslexic person communicate his words on a page. I also have to recognize my long-time editor Al Kingsbury who has helped me for many years in struggling to get my ideas on paper. Without this support, my words would be trapped in my head.

Notes

Introduction

1 Perlita Stroh, "Feeling Lonely? You're Not Alone—And It Could Be Affecting Your Physical Health," CBC News (January 19, 2019), cbc.ca/news/health/national-dealing-with-loneliness-1.4828017.
2 Olga Khazan, "How Loneliness Begets Loneliness," *The Atlantic* (April 6, 2017), theatlantic.com/health/archive/2017/04/how-loneliness-begets-loneliness/521841/.
3 Jackie Tang, Nora Galbraith, and Johnny Truong, "Insights on Canadian Society: Living Alone in Canada," Statistics Canada (March 6, 2019), www150.statcan.gc.ca/n1/pub/75-006-x/2019001/article/00003-eng.htm.
4 Darrell Bricker, "Majority (54%) of Canadians Say Physical Distancing Has Left Them Feeling Lonely or Isolated," Ipsos (April 10, 2020), ipsos.com/en-ca/news-and-polls/Majority-Of-Canadians-Say-Physical-Distancing-Has-Left-Them-Feeling-Lonely-Or-Isolated.
5 David Myers, "The Funds, Friends, and Faith of Happy People," *American Psychologist* 55, no. 1 (2000): 56, doi.org/10.1037/0003-066x.55.1.56.
6 Ed Diener and Martin Seligman, "Very Happy People," *Psychological Science* 13, no. 1 (January 1, 2002): 81–84, doi.org/10.1111/1467-9280.00415.
7 Julianne Holt-Lunstad, Timothy Smith, and J. Bradley Layton, "Social Relationships and Mortality Risk: A Meta-analytic Review," *PLoS Medicine* 7, no. 7 (July 27, 2010): e1000316, doi.org/10.1371/journal.pmed.1000316.

8 Amy Lubik and Tom Kosatsky, "Is Mitigating Social Isolation a Planning Priority for British Columbia (Canada) Municipalities?" BC Centre for Disease Control (September 2019), bccdc.ca/Our-Services-Site/Documents/Social_Isolation_Report_17sept2019.pdf.

9 Julianne Holt-Lunstad, Timothy Smith, and J. Bradley Layton, "Social Relationships and Mortality Risk: A Meta-analytic Review," *PLoS Medicine* 7, no. 7 (July 27, 2010): e1000316, doi.org/10.1371/journal.pmed.1000316.

10 Raheel Mushtaq et al., "Relationship Between Loneliness, Psychiatric Disorders and Physical Health—A Review on the Psychological Aspects of Loneliness," *Journal of Clinical and Diagnostic Research* 8, no. 9 (September 2014), doi.org/10.7860/JCDR/2014/10077.4828.

11 As cited in Emma Seppälä and Marissa King, "Burnout at Work Isn't Just About Exhaustion. It's Also About Loneliness," *Harvard Business Review* (June 29, 2017), hbr.org/2017/06/burnout-at-work-isnt-just-about-exhaustion-its-also-about-loneliness.

12 Nicole K. Valtorta et al., "Loneliness and Social Isolation as Risk Factors for Coronary Heart Disease and Stroke: Systematic Review and Meta-analysis of Longitudinal Observational Studies," *Heart* 102 (April 18, 2016): 1009–16, heart.bmj.com/content/102/13/1009.

13 Tara John, "How the World's First Loneliness Minister Will Tackle 'The Sad Reality of Modern Life,'" *Time* (April 25, 2018), time.com/5248016/tracey-crouch-uk-loneliness-minister/.

14 "Jo Cox Commission on Loneliness," Age UK, ageuk.org.uk/our-impact/campaigning/jo-cox-commission/.

15 Erica Boothby, Margaret Clark, and John Bargh, "Shared Experiences Are Amplified," *Psychological Science* 25, no. 12 (October 1, 2014): 2209–16, doi.org/10.1177/0956797614551162.

16 Bill Howatt, *Stop Hiding and Start Living: How to Say F-it to Fear and Develop Mental Fitness* (Vancouver, BC: Page Two, 2020).

17 Bill Howatt, "Exploring the Relationships Between Perceived Isolation, Loneliness and Resiliency," Workplace Safety & Prevention Services (July 2020), ceohsnetwork.ca/wp-content/uploads/2020/07/exploring-relationships-between-isolation-loneliness-and-resiliency-report.pdf.

Chapter 2: Understand Isolation and Loneliness

1. Karen Rook, "Research on Social Support, Loneliness, and Social Isolation: Toward an Integration," *Review of Personality & Social Psychology* 5 (1984): 239–64, psycnet.apa.org/record/1986-17262-001.
2. "A Portrait of Social Isolation and Loneliness in Canada Today," Angus Reid Institute (June 17, 2019), angusreid.org/social-isolation-loneliness-canada/.
3. Bill Howatt et al., "Why Supporting Employees to Develop Their Coping Skills and Resiliency Is Good Business," Morneau Shepell (August 2017), morneaushepell.com/permafiles/88880/why-supporting-employees-develop-their-coping-skills-and-resiliency-good-business.pdf.
4. Kurtuluş Kaymaz, Umut Eroğlu, and Sayilar Yücel, "Effect of Loneliness at Work on the Employees' Intention to Leave," *Industrial Relations and Human Resources Journal* 16, no. 1 (2014): 38–53, doi.org/10.4026/1303-2860.2014.0241.

Chapter 3: What Causes Social Connections Gaps?

1. Sarah Daniel, "Adult Attachment Patterns and Individual Psychotherapy: A Review," *Clinical Psychology Review* 26, no. 8 (December 2006): 968–84, doi.org/10.1016/j.cpr.2006.02.001.

Chapter 4: The Connection Between Technology and Loneliness

1. Bill Howatt, "Are You Unplugging from Work Each Day?" *Globe and Mail* (August 6, 2019), theglobeandmail.com/business/careers/workplace-award/article-are-you-unplugging-from-work-each-day/.
2. Susan Krauss Whitbourne, "Why Sex Is So Good for Your Relationship," *Greater Good Magazine* (August 3, 2017), greatergood.berkeley.edu/article/item/why_sex_is_so_good_for_your_relationship.
3. See, for example, It's Time to Log Off: itstimetologoff.com/digital-detox-camp-teenagers/.

Chapter 5: How Mental Traps Form

1. Kristin Neff, *Self-Compassion: Stop Beating Yourself Up and Leave Insecurity Behind* (New York: William Morrow, 2011).

2 Shelley Duval and Robert Wicklund, *A Theory of Objective Self-Awareness* (New York: Academic Press, 1972).

3 John Cacioppo et al., "Social Isolation," *Annals of the New York Academy of Sciences* 1231, no. 1 (August 2011): 17-22, doi.org/10.1111/j.1749-6632.2011.06028.x.

4 "Perceived Isolation-Loneliness Effect," Howatt HR Consulting, howatthronline.com/loneliness/.

5 "Choice Theory Psychology," William Glasser International, wglasserinternational.org/courses/professional-development/choice-theory-psychology/. See also chapter 15 in William A. Howatt, *The Human Service Counseling Toolbox: Theory, Development, Technique, and Resources* (Belmont, CA: Brooks/Cole, Cengage Learning, 2000), 126-33, where I explore Glasser's choice theory and reality therapy.

6 Daniel Gilbert and Timothy Wilson, "Miswanting: Some Problems in the Forecasting of Future Affective States," in *Thinking and Feeling: The Role of Affect in Social Cognition*, ed. Joseph Forgas (New York: Cambridge University Press), 178-97, nrs.harvard.edu/urn-3:HUL.InstRepos:14549983.

7 Philip Brickman, Dan Coates, and Ronnie Janoff-Bulman, "Lottery Winners and Accident Victims: Is Happiness Relative?" *Journal of Personality and Social Psychology* 36, no. 8 (1978): 917-27, doi.org/10.1037/0022-3514.36.8.917.

8 Daniel Gilbert, *Stumbling on Happiness* (New York: Vintage Books, 2007).

9 William Glasser, *Choice Theory: A New Psychology of Personal Freedom* (New York: HarperCollins, 1999).

10 David Dozois and Aaron Beck, "Cognitive Schemas, Beliefs and Assumptions," in *Risk Factors in Depression*, ed. Keith Dobson and David Dozois (Cambridge, MA: Elsevier Academic Press, 2008), 121-43, doi.org/10.1016/B978-0-08-045078-0.00006-X.

11 Russ Harris, *ACT Made Simple: An Easy-to-Read Primer on Acceptance and Commitment Therapy* (Oakland, CA: New Harbinger Publications, 2009).

12 James Prochaska, Carlo DiClemente, and John Norcross, "In Search of How People Change: Application to Addictive Behaviors," *American Psychologist* 47, no. 9 (1992): 1102-14, doi.org/10.1037/0003-066X.47.9.1102.

13 Barbara Fredrickson, "The Broaden-and-Build Theory of Positive Emotions," *Philosophical Transactions of the Royal Society B: Biological Sciences* 359, no. 1449 (September 29, 2004): 1367-78, doi.org/10.1098/rstb.2004.1512.

Chapter 6: How to Boost Resiliency

1 David Diamond et al., "The Temporal Dynamics Model of Emotional Memory Processing: A Synthesis on the Neurobiological Basis of Stress-Induced Amnesia, Flashbulb and Traumatic Memories, and the Yerkes-Dodson Law," *Neural Plasticity* 2007 (March 28, 2007): 060803, doi.org/10.1155/2007/60803.
2 Mihaly Csikszentmihalyi, "The Flow Experience and Its Significance for Human Psychology," in *Optimal Experience: Psychological Studies of Flow in Consciousness*, ed. Mihaly Csikszentmihalyi and Isabella Selega Csikszentmihalyi (Cambridge, UK: Cambridge University Press, 1988), 15-35, doi.org/10.1017/CBO9780511621956.002.
3 Paul Eastwick et al., "Mispredicting Distress Following Romantic Breakup: Revealing the Time Course of the Affective Forecasting Error," *Journal of Experimental Social Psychology* 44, no. 3 (May 2008): 800-7, doi.org/10.1016/j.jesp.2007.07.001.
4 Paul Jose, Bee Teng Lim, Fred Bryant, "Does Savoring Increase Happiness? A Daily Diary Study," *Journal of Positive Psychology* 7, no. 3 (May 2012): 176-87, doi.org/10.1080/17439760.2012.671345
5 Robert Emmons and Michael McCullough, "Counting Blessings Versus Burdens: An Experimental Investigation of Gratitude and Subjective Well-Being in Daily Life," *Journal of Personality and Social Psychology* 84, no. 2 (2003): 377-89, doi.org/10.1037/0022-3514.84.2.377.
6 John Mayer and Peter Salovey, "What Is Emotional Intelligence?" in *Emotional Development and Emotional Intelligence: Educational Implications*, ed. Peter Salovey and David J. Sluyter (New York: Basic Books, 1997), 3-34.
7 Albert Mehrabian, *Silent Messages* (Belmont, CA: Wadsworth Publishing, 1971).
8 Bill Howatt, "A 10-Step Routine to Reduce Work Stress One Breath at a Time," *Globe and Mail* (November 23, 2016), theglobeandmail.com/report-on-business/careers/workplace-award/a-10-step-routine-to-reduce-work-stress-one-breath-at-a-time/article33006702/.
9 Bruce Davis, "There Are 50,000 Thoughts Standing Between You and Your Partner Every Day!" *HuffPost* (May 23, 2013), huffpost.com/entry/healthy-relationships_b_3307916.
10 "Mental Illness and Addiction: Facts and Statistics," CAMH, camh.ca/en/driving-change/the-crisis-is-real/mental-health-statistics.

11 As cited in Bill Howatt, "Rewire Your Brain to Think Positively," *Globe and Mail* (November 1, 2017), theglobeandmail.com/report-on-business/careers/workplace-award/rewire-your-brain-to-think-positively/article36798533/. See also Rick Hanson, "Confronting the Negativity Bias," Rick Hanson, Ph.D. (October 16, 2020), rickhanson.net/how-your-brain-makes-you-easily-intimidated/.

12 Michael Merzenich, "Ten Fundamentals of Rewiring Your Brain," The Best Brain Possible (October 4, 2015), thebestbrainpossible.com/the-10-fundamentals-of-rewiring-your-brain/.

13 David Hellerstein, "Neuroplasticity and Depression," *Psychology Today* (July 14, 2011), psychologytoday.com/ca/blog/heal-your-brain/201107/neuroplasticity-and-depression.

14 Richard Widdett, "Neuroplasticity and Mindfulness Meditation" (honours thesis, Western Michigan University, 2014), scholarworks.wmich.edu/honors_theses/2469.

15 As cited in Alina Tugend, "Praise Is Fleeting, but Brickbats We Recall," *New York Times* (March 23, 2012), nytimes.com/2012/03/24/your-money/why-people-remember-negative-events-more-than-positive-ones.html. See also Roy Baumeister et al., "Bad Is Stronger Than Good," *Review of General Psychology* 5, no. 4 (2001): 323-70, doi.org/10.1037/1089-2680.5.4.323.

16 For more on Shawn Achor, see shawnachor.com; for journaling, see Thai Nguyen, "10 Surprising Benefits You'll Get from Keeping a Journal," *HuffPost* (February 13, 2015), huffpost.com/entry/benefits-of-journaling-_b_6648884.

17 As cited in Bill Howatt, "Write Away Your Stress with a Journal," *Globe and Mail* (June 30, 2017), theglobeandmail.com/report-on-business/careers/workplace-award/write-away-your-stress-with-a-journal/article35524429/. See also Heidi Koschwanez, "Expressive Writing and Wound Healing in Older Adults: A Randomized Controlled Trial," *Psychosomatic Medicine* 75, no. 6 (July/August 2013): 581-90, doi.org/10.1097/PSY.0b013e31829b7b2e.

18 Angela Duckworth et al., "From Fantasy to Action: Mental Contrasting with Implementation Intentions (MCII) Improves Academic Performance in Children," *Social Psychological and Personality Science* 4, no. 6 (November 1, 2013): 745-53, doi.org/10.1177/1948550613476307.

19 Nicholas Epley and Juliana Schroeder, "Mistakenly Seeking Solitude," *Journal of Experimental Psychology: General* 143, no. 5 (2014): 1980-99, doi.org/10.1037/a0037323.

20 Erica Boothby, Margaret Clark, and John Bargh, "Shared Experiences Are Amplified," *Psychological Science* 25, no. 12 (October 1, 2014): 2209–16, doi.org/10.1177/0956797614551162.
21 Nicholas Epley, *Mindwise: Why We Misunderstand What Others Think, Believe, Feel, and Want* (New York: Vintage, 2015).
22 John Cacioppo and Stephanie Cacioppo, "The Growing Problem of Loneliness," *The Lancet* 391, no. 10119 (February 3, 2018): 426, doi.org/10.1016/S0140-6736(18)30142-9.
23 "Loneliness Quick Survey," Howatt HR Consulting (2014), howatthronline.com/quicksurveys/lonelinessintro.a5w.
24 Daniel Russell, "UCLA Loneliness Scale (Version 3): Reliability, Validity, and Factor Structure," *Journal of Personality Assessment* 66, no. 1 (1996): 20–40, doi.org/10.1207/s15327752jpa6601_2.

Chapter 7: Framing to Unlock Your Mental Trap

1 Brandon Schmeichel, Adrienne Crowell, and Eddie Harmon-Jones, "Exercising Self-Control Increases Relative Left Frontal Cortical Activation," *Social Cognitive and Affective Neuroscience* 11, no. 2 (February 2016): 282–88, doi.org/10.1093/scan/nsv112.
2 Sonja Lyubomirsky, Kennon Sheldon, and David Schkade, "Pursing Happiness: The Architecture of Sustainable Change," *Review of General Psychology* 9, no. 2 (June 2005): 111–31, doi.org/10.1037/1089-2680.9.2.111.
3 Robert Durham, "Author's Reply," *British Journal of Psychiatry* 166, no. 2 (February 1995): 266–67, doi.org/10.1192/S0007125000183539.

Chapter 8: Unlocking the Mental Trap

1 Matthew Killingsworth and Daniel Gilbert, "A Wandering Mind Is an Unhappy Mind," *Science* 330, no. 6006 (November 12, 2010): 932, doi.org/10.1126/science.1192439.
2 Judson Brewer et al., "Meditation Experience Is Associated with Differences in Default Mode Network Activity and Connectivity," *PNAS* 108, no. 50 (December 13, 2011): 20254–59, doi.org/10.1073/pnas.1112029108.
3 Albert Ellis and Robert Harper, *A New Guide to Rational Living* (Englewood Cliffs, NJ: Prentice-Hall, 1975).
4 William Glasser, *Choice Theory: A New Psychology of Personal Freedom* (New York: HarperCollins, 1999).

5 Dennis Greenberger and Christine Padesky, *Mind over Mood: A Cognitive Therapy Treatment Manual for Clients* (New York: Guilford Press, 1995).
6 Edmund J. Bourne, *The Anxiety & Phobia Workbook*, 7th edition (Oakland, CA: New Harbinger Publications, 2020).
7 William A. Howatt, *My Personal Success Coach: A Guide to Personal Wellness* (Kentville, NS: A Way With Words, 1999).

Chapter 9: The Path to Authentic Connections

1 Jon Kabat-Zinn, *Guided Mindfulness Meditation Practices Series 1* (Boulder, CO: Sounds True, 2005), audio CD.
2 "Examples of Personal Boundaries," Oprah.com (February 5, 2001), oprah.com/spirit/set-your-personal-boundaries/all.
3 For more on The Forgiveness Project, see theforgivenessproject.com.

Chapter 10: Build Authentic Connections with Intention

1 Nicholas Epley and Juliana Schroeder, "Mistakenly Seeking Solitude," *Journal of Experimental Psychology: General* 143, no. 5 (2014): 1980-99, doi.org/10.1037/a0037323.
2 Sonja Lyubomirsky, *The How of Happiness: A New Approach to Getting the Life You Want* (New York: Penguin Books, 2008), 42.
3 Daniel Kahneman and Angus Deaton, "High Income Improves Evaluation of Life but Not Emotional Well-Being," *PNAS* 107, no. 38: 16489-93, doi.org/10.1073/pnas.1011492107.
4 Bernard Van Praag and Paul Frijters, "The Measurement of Welfare and Well-Being: The Leyden Approach," in *Well-Being: The Foundation of Hedonic Psychology*, ed. Daniel Kahneman, Ed Diener, and Norbert Schwarz (New York: Russell Sage Foundation, 1999), 413-33, jstor.org/stable/10.7758/9781610443258.25.
5 Philip Brickman and D.T. Campbell, "Hedonic Relativism and Planning the Good Society," in *Adaptation-Level Theory: A Symposium*, ed. M.H. Appley (New York: Academic Press, 1971), 287-305.
6 Emily Esfahani Smith, "Social Connection Makes a Better Brain," *The Atlantic* (October 29, 2013), theatlantic.com/health/archive/2013/10/social-connection-makes-a-better-brain/280934/.
7 Nattavudh Powdthavee, "Putting a Price Tag on Friends, Relatives, and Neighbours: Using Surveys of Life Satisfaction to Value Social Relationships," *Journal of Socio-Economics* 37, no. 4 (August 2008): 1459-80, doi.org/10.1016/j.socec.2007.04.004.

8 Peter Kolesar, "What Deming Told the Japanese in 1950," in *W. Edwards Deming: Critical Evaluations in Business and Management*, ed. John Wood and Michael Wood (New York: Routledge, 2005), 87–107.
9 John Digman, "Personality Structure: Emergence of the Five-Factor Model," *Annual Review of Psychology* 41, no. 1 (February 1990), 417–40, doi.org/10.1146/annurev.ps.41.020190.002221.
10 Belle Beth Cooper, "Are You an Introvert or an Extrovert? What It Means for Your Career," *Fast Company* (August 21, 2013), fastcompany.com/3016031/are-you-an-introvert-or-an-extrovert-and-what-it-means-for-your-career.
11 Bruce Tuckman, "Developmental Sequence in Small Groups," *Psychological Bulletin* 63, no. 6 (1965), 384–99, doi.org/10.1037/h0022100.

Chapter 11: Loneliness in the Workplace: A Guide for Employers

1 Julianne Holt-Lunstad et al., "Loneliness and Social Isolation as Risk Factors for Mortality: A Meta-analytic Review," *Perspectives on Psychological Science* 10, no. 2 (March 11, 2015), 227–37, doi.org/10.1177/1745691614568352.
2 John Cacioppo and William Patrick, *Loneliness: Human Nature and the Need for Social Connections* (New York: W.W. Norton, 2008).
3 Lea Winerman, "The Mind's Mirror," *Monitor on Psychology* 36, no. 9 (October 2005): 48, apa.org/monitor/oct05/mirror.
4 Stephanie Cacioppo, John Capitanio, and John Cacioppo, "Toward a Neurology of Loneliness," *Psychological Bulletin* 140, no. 6 (November 2014), 1464–504, doi.org/10.1037/a0037618.
5 "The Cost of Loneliness to UK Employers," New Economics Foundation (February 2017), neweconomics.org/uploads/images/2017/02/NEF_COST-OF-LONELINESS_DIGITAL-Final.pdf.
6 S.L. Wagner et al., "Social Support and Supervisory Quality Interventions in the Workplace: A Stakeholder-Centered Best-Evidence Synthesis of Systematic Reviews on Work Outcomes," *International Journal of Occupational and Environmental Medicine* 6, no. 4 (October 2015), 189–204, doi.org/10.15171/ijoem.2015.608.
7 Simon Sinek, *The Infinite Game* (New York: Portfolio, 2019).
8 Poppy Jaman and Garen Staglin, "It's Time to End the Stigma Around Mental Health in the Workplace," World Economic Forum (May 9, 2019), weforum.org/agenda/2019/05/its-time-to-end-the-stigma-around-mental-health-in-the-workplace/.

9 "Mental Health Statistics: Global and Nationwide Costs," Mental Health Foundation, mentalhealth.org.uk/statistics/mental-health-statistics-global-and-nationwide-costs.

10 "Making the Case for Investing in Mental Health in Canada," Mental Health Commission of Canada (2013), mentalhealthcommission.ca/sites/default/files/2016-06/Investing_in_Mental_Health_FINAL_Version_ENG.pdf.

11 Carolyn Dewa, Nancy Chau, and Stanley Dermer, "Examining the Comparative Incidence and Costs of Physical and Mental Health-Related Disabilities in an Employed Population," *Journal of Occupational and Environmental Medicine* 52, no. 7 (July 2010), 758–62, doi.org/10.1097/JOM.0b013e3181e8cfb5. Number of disability cases retrieved from "Mental Illness and Addiction: Facts and Statistics," CAMH, camh.ca/en/driving-change/the-crisis-is-real/mental-health-statistics.

12 "Mental Health in the Workplace," World Health Organization, who.int/mental_health/in_the_workplace/en/.

13 "Why Investing in Mental Health Will Contribute to Canada's Economic Prosperity and to the Sustainability of Our Health Care System," Mental Health Commission of Canada (2014), mentalhealthcommission.ca/sites/default/files/MHStrategy_CaseForInvestment_ENG_0_1.pdf.

14 "The ROI in Workplace Mental Health Programs: Good for People, Good for Business," Deloitte Insights (2019), www2.deloitte.com/content/dam/Deloitte/ca/Documents/about-deloitte/ca-en-about-blueprint-for-workplace-mental-health-final-aoda.pdf.

15 Johanna Badcock et al., "Loneliness in Psychotic Disorders and Its Association with Cognitive Function and Symptom Profile," *Schizophrenia Research* 169, nos. 1–3 (December 2015), 268–73, doi.org/10.1016/j.schres.2015.10.027.

16 "Worry, Gratitude & Boredom: As COVID-19 Affects Mental, Financial Health, Who Fares Better; Who Is Worse?" Angus Reid Institute (April 27, 2020), angusreid.org/covid19-mental-health/.

17 Vivek Murthy, "Work and the Loneliness Epidemic," *Harvard Business Review* (September 26, 2017), hbr.org/cover-story/2017/09/work-and-the-loneliness-epidemic.

18 Matthew Lieberman, *Social: Why Our Brains Are Wired to Connect* (New York: Crown, 2013).

19 As cited in Matthew Kosinski, "When Employees Are Afraid to Speak Up, Organizations Suffer," Recruiter.com (January 3, 2017), recruiter.com/i/when-employees-are-afraid-to-speak-up-organizations-suffer/.

20 Sarah Wang and Eva Karpinski, "Psychological Health in the Workplace," Employment and Social Development Canada (July 14, 2016), canada.ca/en/employment-social-development/services/health-safety/reports/psychological-health.html.
21 Find the Mental Fitness Index (MFI) at "Mental Fitness Training," Howatt HR Consulting, howatthr.com/products-services/mental-fitness-training/.
22 Learn more about Hugr Authentic Connections here: hugr.ca.

Index

Note: Page numbers in italics refer to illustrations

acceptance, self-, 101, 152
Achor, Shawn, 93–94
addiction, 25, 37–38, 63, 120, 153
anger, 151
anxiety, 4, 63, 72, 87, 120, 126, 170
assumptions, 64, 106, 175
attachment theory, 30
authentic (social) connections:
approach to, 2–3, 133–34, 157–58, 159, 182, 195; areas of life for, 143–44; barriers to, 30–32, 76–77; baseline, establishing, 13–15, 163–64; being yourself and, 150, 152, 176; benefits of, 3, 6; boundaries and, 140–42; building and maintaining, 175–80; check-in, 138; as cure for loneliness, 2–3, 6, 9–10; and current circumstances and life stage, 15; evaluation and measurement, 102, 180, 182; expectations and, 150–51, 167, 173, 177; experiments, conducting, 173–75; experiments, example of, 170–72; experiments, preparation for, 173; exposure therapy and, 168–70; facilitation of, 154; false social connections, 36; focus area for finding, 166–67; free choice and, 149–50; fundamentals of, 3, 135–36; genetic need for, 2, 53, 189; happiness and, 3, 159–60; identifying number-one gap, 152; imagining success, 164; inventory of, 142–43, 152, 166; listening and learning, 177; management tips, 145, 147–49; mental health and, 7, 186–88; mental traps and, 144, 147, 168; motivation and, 164–65; nine-step model for creating, 162–63; with people you already know, 156–57; personality types and, 176–77; perspective and, 15; preparation tips, 151–57; as process, 177–78; qualities of authentic and inauthentic relationships, 138–39; recognizing as importance, 101; regret and, 144–45, 166; resiliency and, 102, 103; safety in, 142;

seeking and providing support, 179–80; self-compassion and, 134–35; technology and, 33–34, 193; threats to, 151; value from, 154, 160, 162; values alignment and, 179
awareness: self-awareness, 27, 30, 47, 82, 110, 111–14, 133; social awareness, 82

Band-Aid solutions, 147
Beck, Aaron, 64
behavioural activation system (BAS), 109
behavioural inhibition system (BIS), 109
behaviours. *See* coping behaviours and skills
beliefs, irrational, 127–28
best-case scenarios, 118
Big Five (online personality assessment tool), 176
body language, 83
boundaries, 103, 140–42, 177
Bourne, Edmund J., 126
brain, rewiring, 88–90, 111
breathing, deep, 84–85
broaden-and-build theory, 68
bullying, 51, 185
burnout, 35, 126

Cacioppo, John, 2, 49
catastrophize, 66, 125
change, acceptance of, 104
choice theory, 62–63
cognitive-behavioural approach (CBA): about, 114–15; framing mental traps, 115–17; measurement and, 164; questioning negative thoughts, 120–22; worrying and, 117, 117–18, 120
cognitive hygiene, 86–87

cognitive reframing, 87–88
cognitive schemas, 63–66, 112–13
communication, 83, 148–49, 154–55
compassion: resiliency and, 101; self-compassion, 46–47, 134–35, 152, 153, 195
conflict, 81, 147
contentment, 68
control: self-control, 109; as threat to authentic connections, 151
coping behaviours and skills, 7, 25, 53–54, 59, 60–61, 62–63, 116–17, 118
COVID-19 pandemic, 1–2, 6, 187
critics, 126
curiosity and interest, 68, 105

Dalai Lama, 75
dating apps and services, 155
Deaton, Angus, 159–60
decision making, 83
deep breathing, 84–85
depression, 4, 68–69, 87, 89, 120, 126
disappointment, 68–69
domestic violence, 142
dopamine, 104
dukkha, 154
Durham, Robert, 118

Eastwick, Paul, 77
Edison, Thomas, 150
emotional contagion, 184
emotional intelligence (emotional quotient (EQ)), 79, 81–84
emotional loneliness, 24–25. *See also* loneliness
emotions and feelings: assessment and monitoring of daily emotions, 68, 95, 112; assessment of managing under pressure, 113; being mindful of, 135; check-in, 67; decision

making and, 83; framing mental traps and, 116; negative emotions and mental traps, 66–67, 68–69; removing negative emotions, 124–25; responding to people and, 84
empathy, 82, 83
energy, 77–79, 103
environmental factors, of mental health, 7
expectations, 116, 150–51, 154–55, 167, 173, 177
experiences, shared, 106
exposure therapy, 168–70

failure, 76, 150, 174
false social connections, 36
fear, 57–58, 113, 168–70
feelings. *See* emotions and feelings
fight or flight response, 56–59, 113
finances, and perceived isolation, 51
flow, 72
focused-attention meditation, 91
follow-through, lack of, 151
forgiveness, 147
Frankl, Viktor, 125
free choice, 149–50
fun activities, 104

gender, and perceived isolation, 52
Gilbert, Daniel, 61
Glasser, William, 29, 52–53, 62, 125
goal setting, 96–98
gratitude, 79
grief, 75
group initiatives, 104
guilt and shame, 66, 151

Hanson, Rick, 88
happiness, 3, 103, 104, 106, 111, 121, 159–60

Harris, Russ, 66
health, physical, 7, 103. *See also* mental health
hedonic adaptation, 160
helplessness, learned, 66
Holt-Lunstad, Julianne, 3
Howatt, Bill: *Stop Hiding and Start Living*, 7
Hugr Authentic Connections (app), 193
human gifts, 154

immune neglect, 60–61
indifference, 68
integrity thinking, 101
intention, 75, 99
interest and curiosity, 68, 105
interpersonal skills, 154, 155–56
Inverted U-Model (Yerkes-Dodson law), 72, 73
irrational beliefs, 127–28
isolation: approach to, 8–9, 17–18, 27, 38–39, 195; effects of, 3–4, 120; loneliness and, 9, 17, 22; measurement, 17; measuring workplace risk, 192; as mental health condition, 187–88; moving away from, 24, 29–30; perceived isolation (PI) load, 18–19, 49–56; pervasiveness of, 2, 17; as situational, 23–24; social connections as cure, 2–3, 6, 9–10; subjectiveness and hiddenness of, 22–23; symptoms of, 25–26. *See also* authentic (social) connections; loneliness; mental traps; resiliency; workplace

jealousy, 151
job satisfaction, and perceived isolation, 52
journaling, 93–96, 123
joy, 68

Kabat-Zinn, Jon, 133
Kahneman, Daniel, 159-60
kindness: resiliency and, 102; self-kindness, 134

learned helplessness, 66
Lieberman, Matthew, 189
life purpose, 101
limited thinking, 61-62
listening, 177
logic, faulty, 66
loneliness: approach to, 8-9, 17-18, 27, 38-39, 195; check-in, 26; detection and screening, 21-22, 106-7, 111-12; effects of, 3-4, 120; emotional loneliness, 24-25; as feeling, 105; isolation and, 9, 17, 22; leveraging loneliness drive, 153; loneliness paradox, 36-37; vs. lonely, 19; as mental health condition, 187-88; monitoring, 157; moving away from, 24, 29-30; pervasiveness of, 2, 17; as situational, 23-24; social connections as cure, 2-3, 6, 9-10; social loneliness, 24; vs. solitude, 19; subjectiveness and hiddenness of, 22-23; symptoms of, 25-26. *See also* authentic (social) connections; mental traps; resiliency; workplace
Loneliness Quick Survey, 106
lying, 151
Lyubomirsky, Sonja, 159

management, self-, 82
manager-employee relationship, 52
Mayer, John, 79
meditation, 91, 123-24. *See also* mindfulness
mental contrast, 97

mental fitness: within mental health, 7; resiliency and, 77, 101-2, 107-8
Mental Fitness Index (MFI), 192
mental health: four pillars of, 6-7; as personal value, 110-11; social connections and, 186-88; statistics on, 185; staying safe, 46; workplace and, 184-86, 187
mental illness: loneliness and, 120; perceived isolation and, 52; prevalence of, 185, 187; stress and negative thinking, 72, 89
mental traps: approach to, 43-44, 69, 109-10, 123-24, 128-29; authentic connections and, 144, 147, 168; causes of, 53; check-ins, 45, 54; and choosing thoughts and emotions, 124-25; cognitive-behavioural approach for, 114-18, 120-22; coping behaviours and, 53-54, 60-61, 62-63, 116-17; fight or flight response and, 56-59; and frequency, duration, and intensity of unwanted thoughts, 47, 49; Glasser on basic needs and, 52-53; happiness framework and, 111; irrational beliefs and, 127-28; long-term effects, 44-45, 46; monitoring emotions and, 68; negative emotions and, 66-67, 68-69; perceived isolation and, 49-52, 54-56; personality and, 125-26; self-awareness and, 47, 111-14; self-compassion and, 46-47; self-control and, 109; staying safe, 46; thoughts and, 59-66; unlocking, 44, 45-46, 71, 123-29; values framework and, 110-11
micro-social touches, 106

mindfulness, 81, 92–93, 123–24. *See also* meditation
mirror neurons, 184
mistakes, admitting to, 156
miswanting, 60
motivation, 101, 110, 164–65
Murthy, Vivek H., 188

neuroplasticity, 89, 111

online peer groups, 105
outward focus, 105

paradox, loneliness, 36–37
perceived isolation, 18–19, 49–52, 54–56
Perceived Isolation-Loneliness Effect survey, 51
perfection and perfectionists, 104, 126
persistence, 105
personal connections, 153
personality, 125–26, 176–77
perspective, 15, 95, 114–15
pets, 104
physical health, 7, 103. *See also* mental health
plans, 162–63
pleasure, 104
positivity, rewiring brain for, 88–90
predictions, future, 118
present, being, 102
Pressman, Sarah, 4
prospect theory, 94
psychological safety, in workplace, 23–24, 58–59, 189, 191–93
purpose, life, 101

quality world pictures, 53

reality therapy, 29
reciprocation, 148, 178
regret, 144–45
rejection, in relationships, 152
relationship management, 82. *See also* authentic (social) connections
resiliency: approach to, 71, 107–8; benefits of, 7, 9, 77; cognitive hygiene and, 86–87; cognitive reframing and, 87–88; deep breathing and, 84–85; emotional intelligence and, 79, 81–84; energy drains and boosters, 77–79; goal setting and, 96–98; isolation vs. loneliness and, 22; journaling and, 93–96; meditation and, 91; mindful visualization and, 92–93; rewiring brain for positivity and, 88–90; stress and, 72–75; tips for, 99, 101–7; training, 75–77
respect, mutual, 3
responses, to others, 156
restorative justice, 162

safety: in mental health, 46; in relationships, 142
Salovey, Peter, 79
scenarios, best- and worst-case, 118
seclusion, 19
self-acceptance, 101, 152
self-awareness, 27, 30, 47, 82, 110, 111–14, 133
self-compassion, 46–47, 101, 134–35, 152, 153, 195
self-control, 109
self-kindness, 134
self-management, 82
self-perceptions, negative, 66
self-talk: faulty self-talk, 66, 69; positive self-talk, 152

shame and guilt, 66, 151
shared experiences, 106
showing up, 102-3
Sinek, Simon, 185
sleep, 105
SMART goals, 97
social activities, 150, 153, 156
social awareness, 82
social connection practice, 155
social connections gaps: barriers to connection, 30-32, 76-77; coping strategies, 60-61; effects of, 4; hedonic adaptation and, 160. *See also* authentic (social) connections; loneliness; mental traps
social distancing, 1-2
social loneliness, 24. *See also* loneliness
social media, 33-34, 36-37, 102
social skills, 34-36
solitude, 19
spontaneity, 155
stories, telling, 156
stress, 4, 72-75, 84, 93-96
success, imagining, 164
support, seeking and providing, 179-80

talents, sharing, 104
teams, and perceived isolation, 52
technology: check-in, 38; compulsive behaviour and, 37-38; for creating social connections, 193; false social connections and, 36; loneliness paradox, 36-37; role in social connections and loneliness, 33-34, 38; social skills and, 34-36; unplugging from, 102
thoughts: being mindful of negative thoughts, 135; check-ins, 65, 121; choice theory and, 61-62; cognitive hygiene, 86-87; cognitive reframing, 87-88; framing mental traps and, 116; immune neglect and, 60-61; influence on actions, 30, 59-60; irrational beliefs, 127-28; miswanting, 60; negative cognitive schemas and faulty self-talk, 63-66, 105, 109-10, 112-13, 134; questioning negative thoughts, 120-22; removing negative thoughts, 124-25; rewiring brain for positivity, 88-90; self-destructive thinking, 125
time, for relationships, 178
toxic relationships, 154
Tuckman, Bruce, 177

UCLA Loneliness Scale, 106
United Kingdom, 4, 184
unplugging, from technology, 102

values, 110-11, 179
victims, 126
violence, domestic, 142
visualization, mindful, 92-93

well-being journal, 95-96
Winfrey, Oprah, 140
WOOP goal-setting model, 97
workplace: boundaries for work, 103; check-in, 188; emotional contagion and, 184; leadership's role, 188-89; loneliness effects in, 183-84; mental health and, 184-86; perceived isolation and, 51, 52; psychological safety in, 23-24, 58-59, 189, 191-93; social connections and mental health, 186-88
worry and worriers, *117*, 117-18, 120, 126
worst-case scenarios, 118

Yerkes-Dodson law (Inverted U-Model), *72, 73*

zone, being in the, 72

About the Author

Known as one of Canada's top experts in mental health issues in the workplace, Dr. Bill Howatt is the president of Howatt HR. Bill's life has not been an easy path. He understands the daily struggle of being a human being. Bill has had some major setbacks that have challenged his resiliency, such as being adopted, failing grade two, and living with a mental illness. If it were not for his positive experience at Acadia University, he may not be where he is today. He has 30-plus years' experience in mental health and addictions counselling, HR, and leadership. He is a regular columnist for the *Globe and Mail* and the *Chronicle Herald*, an instructor for the University of New Brunswick, and the author of over 400 articles and 40 books.

billhowatt.com
howatthr.com

Work with Dr. Bill Howatt

Dr. Bill Howatt is available to speak to your team or company on the topics of mental fitness, resiliency, and loneliness.

billhowatt.com
Twitter: @billhowatt
LinkedIn: /howatthr

Dr. Bill Howatt is the president of Howatt HR, a human resources firm focused on psychological health and safety. Howatt HR's purpose is to support employers, leaders, and employees to reduce mental harm and promote mental health in the workplace. Hire Howatt HR to assist with shaping and strengthening culture, building psychologically safe leaders, and boosting employees' mental fitness.

howatthr.com

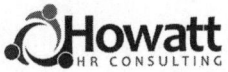

Looking for Additional Resources to Feel Connected?

Hugr Authentic Connections is a mental wellness app designed to help people feel connected. Through the self-guided digital program, individuals can measure their level of social connection, discover how to build and maintain authentic connections, and regularly share how they're feeling with those closest to them.

Hover the camera of your phone over the QR code below to access a free version of Hugr Authentic Connections.

hugr.ca

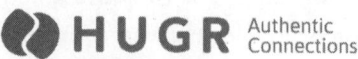